WHAT THE
Fork?

The
Secret Cause
of Disease

GINA BONANNO-LEMOS

What The Fork?

The Secret Cause of Disease

The content of this book is for general instruction only. Each person's physical, emotional, and spiritual condition is unique. The instruction in this book is not intended to replace or interrupt the reader's relationship with a physician or other professional. Please consult your doctor or other health professional of your choice for matters pertaining to your specific health and diet.

To contact the author:

www.360HealthConnection.com

ISBN-10: 0692639829
ISBN-13: 978-0692639825

Library of Congress Control Number: 2016905329
360 Health Connection, Yorba Linda, CA

Printed in the United States of America

*This book is dedicated
to my incredible children*

You are my sunshine!

Foreward

By Ocean Robbins,
CEO, The Food Revolution Network

What you eat is very personal. After all, it literally becomes you.

Throughout most of the history of our species, we've eaten whatever we could get ahold of. Getting enough calories to survive was the goal.

But in the modern world, that's changed. We now have access to a vast array of tastes, textures, and cuisines. In the modern world, the fundamental goal of food has come to be driven by commerce, pleasure, and convenience.

I love to see people make a good living, and I love to see people have more ease and joy in their lives. But the tragic reality is that the food norms of the modern world turn out to be sickening and even killing us.

Fortunately, we have people like Gina Bonanno-Lemos here to point the way to another possibility. Here to show us that we don't have to be sick and allergic and overweight, and that health doesn't need to be elusive.

Gina's message is entertaining, and her book is a delight to read. But don't be deceived – it's also very serious. Like any good book, it's a pleasure to read. And like the best of books, it will give you something that could improve the quality of your life.

Gina has lived out loud, and in these pages, she'll take you on a richly illustrated journey that is hers. But she'll also share a story that could be any of ours. And through her pain, and her transformation, there are lessons that could bring greater health to millions.

Enjoy!

Contents

Introduction

Who among us hasn't been touched by disease and illness? And who doesn't know at least a half dozen people taking one or more prescription medications?

All of us have either been directly or indirectly affected by the ravages of heart disease, cancer, or diabetes, and we all know people who suffer with other ailments that greatly reduce quality of life and/or mobility and cognitive function. What's worse is that these life-taking and life-altering afflictions know no boundaries and don't discriminate. They affect people of all ages, all social and economic classes, all races and creeds, and all levels of education.

Yes, people are dying. Friends and family members are dying. And those who aren't dying are getting sicker and becoming more depleted each day.

This is probably not news to you because mainstream media does a great job of terrifying everyone, almost daily, with statistics about obesity and disease rates while offering little hope or promoting the latest diet craze to "lose ten pounds in ten days."

Workout gurus tell you that you just need to eat less and exercise more, but the general consensus is that there's not a whole lot you can do about your physical status. It's just the way it is, and that's just what happens when you get older.

Pharmaceutical companies advise that you pop some pills and hope that you're one of the "lucky" ones, while they push their marked-up inventory at every commercial break offering relief for your symptoms.

All the while the government claims that there still aren't any cures for the diseases with the highest mortality rates. They just can't seem to figure out the causes, no matter how much money pours in for research.

Millions walk for the cure or run for the cause, and pink ribbons adorn every product imaginable. It's BIG business and has raked in billions in donations, yet there are still no answers.

But what if it's all BS? What if you, and everyone you know, have been lied to about what's really causing all of this disease and illness? And what if there's an easy way to cure or even prevent these ailments, even the life-threatening ones, by means of a sane and simple protocol?

What they don't tell you–indeed, –what they *won't* tell you– is that we are not victims of our genetics or age. You will never hear them tell the truth—that *you* hold the power to control your health outcome up to 95% of the time[1-3].

They'll never tell you that cutting out just one type of food can literally mean the difference between life and death!

When I learned the truth, it turned my beliefs and perceptions upside down, and I soon discovered that I had been fed a load of crap my entire life, both literally and figuratively. And it started with my conversation over coffee with a friend.

Little did I know that this coffee date would inspire the most profound transformation in my entire existence and radically alter the trajectory of my life. It was one of several turning points over the course of a year that changed my life and health in unimaginable ways.

For that reason this book is far more than a nutrition guide or narrative about how I went about healing my body and getting my life back. Instead it is a story of spiritual inspiration and a reckoning of the soul.

I invite you to come along with me as I share the story of my healing as well as information that has been concealed from you—Information that has the power to change your life for the better.

Throughout these pages you'll see the names of people who are heroes, yet you may have never heard of them before. After I made the decision to heed the advice of these experts, some of whom are considered to be on the fringe of our society, I experienced astonishing health results. These leaders in the health movement acted as my guides, and they led me to a place of physical, emotional, and spiritual health that I never believed was possible.

Now it's your turn!

Imagine looking in the mirror and seeing a younger version of yourself each morning.

Imagine having surplus energy to truly enjoy every moment of every day.

INTRODUCTION

Imagine living each day free from physical and emotional pain and finally being in control of your health and happiness.

It happened *for* and to me, and it can happen for you too!

1

So Sick

My life had taken a 180 degree turn, and I no longer recognized myself. I began to view the people around me differently as well, and I began to question everything that I thought I knew.

Sound like a bad thing? In reality, it was the best thing that ever happened *for* me, and it gave my life purpose once again.

It began during a time when my husband and I were coming out of a financial tailspin. This was after the real estate market crash and after less than ethical business partners left us with two failed businesses and completely depleted retirement accounts.

I can joke about it now to some degree. I tell my husband that those were the years of our "non-profit" businesses.

Needing to get back on our financial feet, my husband and I went back to what we knew best and what had made us money consistently–real estate and mortgages. I jumped into the ice-cold water with both feet, experiencing that energy-sucking feeling of returning to a job that makes it possible to feed your family but does nothing to feed your soul.

I worked day and night on building my real estate blog and online presence to over 10,000 views monthly. Within 6 months I was bringing in so many leads that I had to hire additional agents to help with clients all over Southern California. By all accounts it was a success, but even with this "success" my spirit was withering.

I was miserable. I felt trapped and dead inside. I knew in the depths of my being that I was not meant to work in the real estate industry. I *had* a purpose to fulfill in life, but what was it? Yes, real estate was a way to pay bills, and I liked meeting new people, but I felt as if the very air that I breathed was being sucked out of me every single day. And I was sick– God, was I sick–and exhausted beyond belief. This was nothing new for me, though.

As a child I missed tons of school every year due to allergies, asthma, colds and the flu. A few absences, I will admit, were because I forgot to set the VCR for *General Hospital*, so I had a horrible "stomach ache" and needed to go home to find out what happened to Luke and Laura.

Anyhooo, I was really sick *all the time*! And, unlike most people, as I got older it got worse. My late teens and twenties were plagued by chronic sinus infections that would last for weeks on end, until I'd finally give up from lack of sleep and get a prescription for antibiotics. These ongoing bouts of sinus hell became like a menstrual cycle. I actually began tracking when they would hit, and I would let people know that I couldn't go out that week or weekend because I would be sick at that time. They'd look at me like I needed to put the crack pipe down, and I know it sounded crazy, but it was true, and it sucked!

Doctors even treated me like some kind of freak of nature who needed to be sized for a plastic bubble like John Travolta (Yeah, I'm a child of the 70's. What can I say?). I remember distinctly, when I was SO over my allergies in my twenties, that I decided to go for it, and get allergy immunizations. I went to the allergist's office and had the scratch test performed on my back. This is the first part of their testing process in which they draw boxes on your skin and then scratch you with a wooden stick that has a bit of each allergen on the tip. I squirmed and fidgeted like crazy as I lay there for the required twenty minute period waiting for the results to appear in the form of welts. The scratch test revealed that I was extremely allergic to everything under the sun (I could have told them that and saved a co-pay), so they requested that I undergo further testing via a blood sample to narrow down how many types of trees and grasses I was allergic to.

On my second visit I waited in a room for my results. I heard the nurse mention my name and inform the doctor of my room number. The door was cracked, and as the doctor moved closer I could tell from his slow and deliberate pace that he was reviewing a medical chart. He stopped when he reached the door, and I could see the shadow of his shoe protruding through the opening. The door began to open ever so slowly until I could see a partial profile of his face. His hand slid across the wood surface and I could see that his body was angled away from the entrance, as if he suspected that the door had been rigged with a bomb and that he might find it necessary to sprint and barrel roll to safety at any moment. This struck me as odd because most doctors simply grab the door knob, knock out of courtesy, and then barge in as if they own the joint. And well, technically, I guess they kinda do. I tried to hide it, but I'm quite certain that my face mirrored his expression of bewilderment and fear because at this point I was thoroughly convinced that I had some rare disease and needed to be rushed to the hospital immediately. Now facing me, he took a few cautious steps into the room, peered at me over the rim of his glasses and remarked, "You're a highly allergic young lady, aren't you?". Again, I could have told them that.

As I grew older into my thirties, my health continued to dictate every part of my life. I declined invitations for parties and holiday events because I knew that if the host had pets or someone had a cold or flu and I *did* attend, it would mean weeks of downtime and more meds. So I stayed home, isolated and wondering whether I would ever be able to live a normal life and be like everyone else.

These chronic illnesses even affected my career choices. At one point, after having fallen in love with weight lifting in high school, I considered becoming a personal trainer. Then I realized that I might have to meet with clients in their homes. This prospect scared the hell out of me. Why? Was it because they might be serial killers, luring young women into their den of death? Nope. It was the fear that they might have a pet, maybe even a cat, whose dander floated about for months, waiting for my allergy-ridden body to land on. I would imagine a scenario something like the following:

As I walk in to greet my client, his smiling face turns into that of a grinning clown. The suspender-wearing, floppy-shoed ogre throws his red, cul-de-sac hairline back and roars with evil laughter. Over his shoulder I catch a glimpse of a giant hair-ball the size of a tumbleweed rolling in my direction. I turn and run, only to trip (as all of the uncoordinated female characters do in horror flicks).

I scramble back onto my feet, and as I dash for the door, I glance over my shoulder. It's coming ever so slowly yet seemingly gaining on me at lightning speed (as all of the menacing creatures do in scary movies). Fumbling with the lock and knob, I manage to fling the door open just in time. Cool air hits my cheek, offering a welcome reminder that I'm close to safety.

I sprint to my car and drop my keys just as I'm approaching (you know why). After retrieving them from the ground, I push a button, but I hear only one beep. Damn it! In my panic I've pushed the lock button. I hit unlock and jump in. After I lock the car door, I screech out of the driveway in reverse like Mario Andretti with dementia. Once on the street I slam the gear shift into drive, and a lone tear streams down my cheek.

Finally, when I reach a safe distance, I glance in the rearview mirror. With the hair-ball nowhere in sight, I say a prayer of thanks for escaping the house of hell. Just then I catch a glimpse of the most terrifying sight. "It can't be!", I cry, "I ran as fast as I could." Surely this couldn't be happening, but it has. I stare blankly into the mirror, knowing that the next few weeks of my life are over, as a lone cat hair sits on my shoulder, mocking me. My mouth widens as I scream in horror, "AAAAAAAAAH!"

And scene.

2

You Dropped
A Bomb On Me

So back to reality and on with my life-altering, earth shattering-event.

It was October, and I had made plans to meet my friend Sandi for coffee. Sandi was a lot of fun to hang out with and it had been far too long since we'd seen each other or had a lengthy conversation, so I was excited to catch up. We originally became acquainted during a brief business venture with which I became involved, and we had hit it off immediately. We shared a background in real estate and an interest in health. Twenty-six years my senior, Sandi was someone to be admired. She was as sharp as could be, full of energy, and always learning a new skill and taking up new hobbies.

After arriving at Starbucks and greeting each other, we got in line to order our drinks. When our names were called I picked up my quad shot cappuccino and Sandi, her herbal tea. I added some half-and-half to my cup and offered the pitcher to Sandi, who declined. Finding it odd that she didn't put anything into her drink I asked, "You don't want anything in your tea?" to which Sandi replied, "No. I don't drink dairy anymore."

I shrugged and assumed that she was lactose-intolerant. After we found an open table and sat down, I asked her when she had stopped drinking dairy. That's when Sandi explained that she had become a vegan about a year earlier after her doctor ran some tests and had diagnosed her as having the beginning stages of heart disease. I was shocked. I mean, here I was with someone who was always physically active and, to my knowledge, had a healthy diet. And yet, she was developing heart disease? I was even more shocked to hear that she had gone the vegan route. What the hell was going on? Was I in an alter universe? Vegans were nuts. Weren't they those croc-wearing, tree-hugging crazies who didn't understand the fundamentals of nutrition?

I had studied nutrition and fitness. I had studied everything I could get my hands on in a book or magazine for more than twenty years, or at least I thought I had. I had been lifting weights since I was fifteen years old and *knew* that we needed animal protein. We couldn't possibly be healthy or live without it. What was she thinking?

Then Sandi told me how she went home from that doctor's appointment and picked up an unread book that she had had for years. Apparently someone had given it to her as a gift, but she threw it on a bookshelf and had never given it a second thought until her diagnosis. It was Dr. Caldwell Esselstyn's book titled, *Prevent and Reverse Heart Disease.* That book, as Sandi went on to say, had changed and possibly saved her life. She had gone vegan "cold turkey," throwing out or giving away nearly every animal product in her fridge, freezer, and pantry. About six months later she returned to her doctor for a follow-up examination. After declining his prescription medication, which made her feel tired and caused her to gain weight, her cardiologist was surprised to report that her numbers had decreased and that she had reversed her incipient heart disease.

I couldn't believe what I was hearing, and I was intrigued. I must admit that, had the story come from someone I didn't respect, I doubt that I would have been so open to the information.

I listened intently as Sandi went on to tell me that her boyfriend had successfully reversed his diabetes by following her lead and adopting a plant-based diet as well. He had also lost more than twenty-five pounds within six months without any extra effort and no longer needed his daily medication.

Okay, now Sandi had me. Not quite at hello, but she had me,

and I wanted to learn more. My friend advised that I read *The China Study* and watch a documentary called *Forks Over Knives*.

Then she said something I'll never forget. It was a soul-reckoning moment that shook me to the core. Without an ounce of personal judgment directed at me, Sandi said, "I just don't understand how animal lovers can eat animals. I mean, they all have little personalities and feel pain."

WOW, that one innocent observation cut deep. *I* was an animal lover. I had loved all animals for my entire life. I was the person who drove by farms and made mooing and neighing noises while my family made fun of me.

How had this simple yet profound concept eluded me for forty-some years? I loved animals, yet I was *choosing* to eat them up to three times every day. Apparently I had some soul-searching to do.

We said our goodbyes later that morning, and I drove off replaying our conversation in my head. Could Sandi's regimen possibly help *me* feel better? Could it be this great when I'd never heard anything positive about a vegan diet before? I had a sense that something big was coming. I don't know how else to describe it other than as a pleasant anxiety.

3

Here You Come Again

What was it, I wondered, with all this vegan garbage? It kept popping up in my life. I remembered watching an Oprah show where people talked about the pros and cons of vegan diets. All of Oprah's employees had gone vegan for a month and they shared their health and weight-loss success stories with the audience.

Oprah's producers had even found a "beef-production plant," as they called it, which allowed their cameras and Lisa Ling in to view their procedures. Interestingly, they mentioned that every other production plant they contacted had declined their request to film what went on behind the scenes. I remember wondering why these plants wouldn't want their operations to be filmed. I mean, it's normal to kill animals for food, right? Was it really *that* bad? I quickly dismissed these thoughts when one of the Oprah show's guests made the following statement:

"Animals have one bad day." His comment stuck with me and provided justification for my choices. I liked him. He seemed logical and didn't challenge my existing views.

I also thought back to a couple of conversations about the macrobiotic diet. I knew two people who had cured their cancer by using nothing but this food protocol. One of them, Mina Dobic, who subsequently became a macrobiotic teacher and healer, had been given only weeks to live, having been told by her doctors that there was no cure for her stage-four condition. Mina lived across the street from my aunt, and their daughters were friends. My aunt had shared Mina's miraculous story with me years before my conversation with Sandi, and I had taken the time to research the macrobiotic diet. What I found was that it's similar to a vegan diet in many ways. Although it does allow for the periodic consumption of a few types of fish, all other animal products are strictly prohibited. At the time I thought it was interesting, but I wasn't interested enough to dig any deeper.

I know, though, that when things keep showing up in your life, whether good or bad, there's a reason for it. There's a lesson that we're meant to learn. And the greatest lessons of all can come in the form of a challenge placed at our feet. This is one of life's greatest gifts if we choose to unwrap it. However, when we dismiss recurring themes as coincidence or bad luck, we fail to discover our true purpose or to become the highest and best form of ourselves.

Knowing this, I picked up a copy of *The China Study* a few weeks after my meeting with Sandi. I took it along on a trip to Yosemite and read it from cover to cover during our week-long vacation. Being a stats geek, I lost myself in the data and case studies.

What I read was shocking. Could it really be true that cancer and other diseases are caused by our consumption of animal protein? The research was solid, convincing, and impressive . The book presented multiple studies across several continents and included clinical data on both animals and humans, completed by numerous physicians and scientists.

In my gut I knew that the information had to be accurate, and I knew also that I had to make a change. But did I really want to?

4

I Can't Go
For That

The one positive thing about constantly fighting illnesses (always looking for the silver lining here) is that you tend to be more open-minded to alternative treatments and out-of-the-box thinking (and by "box", I mean conventional Western medicine). Like most chronically ill people, I thought that I had tried everything. I went the traditional medical route for more than twenty years; I allowed doctors to jab me with needles every week for allergy shots; I had sinus surgery to remove nasal polyps; I tried every pill, potion, and nasal spray known to man, and I changed my diet as appropriate, when the newest medical research was published in magazines and made the news. When the traditional methods failed me I turned to an alternative medicine doctor, with whom I worked for more than 10 years, taking whole food supplements and trying nearly every new procedure and treatment he offered. Although he was able to remedy a few of my issues, I remained sick and tired. So how would a vegan diet help me when everything else had failed? Surely, if a vegan diet could cure me of all my problems, a doctor would have mentioned it somewhere along the way.

It just didn't seem plausible that an exclusively plant-based diet would have any kind of positive effect on my health, and I would be miserable in the process, so what was the point? And I thought I knew what a vegan diet was, and it didn't sound appealing at all: you ate tofu and salads everyday and sang "Kumbaya" around a campfire at night, right?

Logically, I knew that I must be missing something, a piece of the puzzle, but was this puzzle even real, or just another false hope? My biggest question was, how in the world was I going to get any protein and enough calories eating nothing but plants?

Like so many people, I didn't have all the answers when I first ventured down this path, and I didn't have a clue about where to start. I recognize now that I wasn't completely committed to making this change; otherwise I could have turned to my friend Sandi for advice. It wasn't until it became an emotional issue for me that I made the decision to commit myself 100%.

So here I was, half in and half out as in a game of Hokie Pokie.

I was "cutting back" on animal products, but I found plenty of excuses for not cutting out animal protein entirely.

My top excuse? My family will never go for this.

I'll never forget when I first mentioned a vegan diet to my husband. It was shortly after I read *The China Study*, and his exact words were "F**k that" (and, no, it wasn't "Fork"). Not exactly inspiring and supportive.

Then there was my teenage daughter. Oh brother, was she a tough nut to crack! She said unequivocally, "I am not giving up meat."

Luckily my son was already living on his own. Otherwise he probably would have helped them declare me insane and fit me for a straight-jacket.

Given the resounding sentiments of my husband and daughter, I told my friend Sandi that I didn't think I would be able to make a complete change to a plant-based diet. Although I was excluding animal products from my lunch, I hadn't been able to forego turkey bacon at breakfast, and I *had* to cook some sort of meat for dinner, lest I be served with divorce papers for "irreconcilable food differences" or reported to CPS for failure to provide proper nourishment.

I remember thinking that if I did this, if I made this major change, I'd be doing it on my own. I'd have to watch everyone around me eating the foods that I'd always loved, and I'd be cooking multiple meals for dinner.

And, oh, how I love my food! My love for food is known far and wide, even earning me nicknames such as "the spider" and "food whore." I've got quite a "rep" as well with my Aunt Debi. She has said that when she's old and bedridden she wants my cousin to bring her marijuana for pain because she's younger and "will know where to get it." And she wants me to bring her food because I know "where to get all the best food" and the "best items on the menu."

So what was I to do? I had a husband and daughter who were ready to revolt, and I wasn't completely sold on the idea of giving up the main portion of my meals anyway, so I muddled along with my meatless lunches and pretended that I was trying to go vegan.

5

Desperate But Not Serious

January arrived and I was in the midst of my second lung infection in two months. This one was scarier than the last. My lungs were almost completely shutting down on me, and my inhaler wasn't working. If it did, I got about fifteen minutes of relief before I'd start wheezing and coughing again. I visited my holistic doctor, who gave me new supplements and a nebulizer to open up my lungs. He said that I should use it every four hours, but I couldn't go more than one to two hours without feeling as though I were being suffocated. The infection lasted for a full three weeks, during which time I slept propped up on pillows and woke constantly shaking as I struggled to take in oxygen. This episode was bad and, as usual, left me unable to take care of all of my responsibilities.

What was it going to take for me to get healthy? I felt like death warmed over (as my grandmother used to say), I was completely wiped out all the time, and I wasn't getting any younger. As a matter of fact, I had just met with a specialist to have my hormone levels tested. She informed me that I had officially entered the perimenopausal stage of life. "That's just faaaantastic," I said to myself. Well, at least that explained the unusual weight gain around my waist over the previous eighteen months, and I finally understood why my extremely swollen face made me barely recognizable in photos. And the best part of all? It was only going to get worse from here on out. Oh yay (she said, with a boat load of sarcasm)!

I realized that this must be what women bitched about as they got older.

I had reduced my portion sizes at meals, and I had even added a full-blown cardio workout to my weight lifting routine, all to no avail. And it wasn't as though I was eating unhealthy food. I mean, at our meals we had lean meats like turkey, chicken or fish, and we rarely ate beef and almost *never* pork. I also insisted that everyone in the family have some sort of fruit or a vegetable with each meal, and we consumed only whole grains–no simple carbohydrates that would turn into sugar. So what the hell!? What more could I do?

With my lung infection finally behind me in February, I accepted an invitation from Sandi to meet for lunch at a vegan restaurant. I was scared.

We met at The Loving Hut, one of her "favorites." We made small talk as I browsed through the menu. I was only half listening to what Sandi was saying because my inner dialogue sounded like this:

"Oh my God, how in the hell am I going to choke this down without making faces?"

"Please, please, don't let it taste like crap."

"Oh well, I can always eat when I get home. I'll just take a few bites and tell Sandi that I'm not that hungry and that I'm gonna take it home for later."

Feeling completely lost and looking for some help, I asked Sandi what her favorite menu item was. She said, "Oh, I don't know. Everything they make is great." Then she rattled off about eight to ten different items that she had eaten before.

"Well hell," I thought, "that doesn't help me at all."

So I was on my own. I kept searching the menu, and found something called Hainam Grilled Rice. I remember thinking, "Okay, I know what rice is, and I know what grilled means. I guess the Hainam part will be a surprise. Hopefully the rice will be enough to fill me up and this dish won't have some sort of weird vegan sauce on it."

Our lunch was served, and it actually looked... good. I took a bite of the rice first. "Hmmm, that *is* good," I thought. Then for the real test. I cut a piece of the chicken-looking substance and, with trepidation, placed it on my tongue. The flavor was pleasing, so I began to chew, expecting it to be some creepy, rubbery fake meat. But no. Wait a minute; hold the phone; shut the front door. It was, dare I say, delicious, and it had the consistency of a real chicken breast!

Needless to say, I cleaned my plate and even dipped my rice and "chicken" in the sauce that came with the meal. It too, was aaaawsome (emphasis on the 'a' and said in a tone, two octaves higher than normal).

I went home and told my family all about my experience. They weren't impressed, but I kept thinking, "Wow. If I could have meals like that three times a day, I'd totally go vegan and never miss animal meat."

I marched on, still considering a vegan way of life, but not yet embracing it. I tried a myriad varieties of "fakin' bacon" for breakfast. They ranged in flavor from disturbing to disgusting, and as I tired of faux hot dogs, soy lunch "meats" and salads for lunch, I did what any sensible and intelligent person would do. I turned to the all-knowing Google.

I wasn't quite sure what to Google at first, so I started with the obvious "vegan." This didn't yield the kind of results in which I was interested, but I kept trying, and as one website led me to another I gathered intel. That was when I found the images and information that would change everything . I had discovered exactly what I needed to move this idea from my head to my heart and make it real for me.

6

What You Don't Know

They say that a picture is worth a thousand words, and how true those words are. A few pictures turned the topic of vegansim into my mission. I was no longer kicking the tires. I was now behind the wheel, speeding away with the pink slip in my hand and running every red light in town.

It was those few photos of desperate eyes silently pleading for mercy and begging for salvation that transformed my resistance to resolve.

Those pictures were of animals, some in their last moments, some in the *worst* moments of their lives. Now I know that you must be thinking, "Well, isn't the last moment of their lives automatically the worst?" I can tell you without a doubt that for the majority of these animals it's NOT EVEN CLOSE to their worst moment.

What I've witnessed in photos and videos is almost too horrific for words.

I shudder when I think back on how I thoughtlessly ate whatever sounded good to me. Maya Angelou's words came to mind; "When you know better, you do better." I knew that what I was witnessing in these photos had to stop. I couldn't be a part of it any longer.

I kept asking myself how I had lived for so many years in the dark. I guess that I had always had certain images in my head. You know, the visuals that commercials have pounded into our memory banks, like the ones of "happy cows" and Old McDonald's Farm, or the ones of animals roaming in a grassy meadow, on acres and acres of land, with fresh air and blue skies all around.

I bought into it. I believed that these animals were on a pasture somewhere lying in the sun, enjoying their lives, and communing with their fellow creatures. I believed that the people who raised these animals did so with love and care. I believed that these caretakers in some way appreciated the animals for forfeiting their lives so that farmers could make a living. I also imagined that the animal's lives were taken with as little pain as possible, that they were "put to sleep" and euthanized like our beloved pets. Oh how wrong I was about absolutely everything!

What I didn't know, what I didn't have a clue about, was the existence of factory farms. I had never even heard the term before.

So what *is* a factory farm? Factory farms[1], officially called Confined Animal Feeding Operations (CAFO), are essentially hell on earth for animals–a place where animals are literally born to die. This is where animals are mass-produced and treated as nothing more than a consumer product. Like an object rather than a living being, they are thought of as some*thing*, rather than someone. And the name of the game is speed for profit, so the faster these "things" can be produced and packaged, the more money the manufacturers make.

Long gone are the days of small farmers who tended to their animals and interacted with them daily. Animals are now housed on top of each other, quite literally in the case of egg-laying hens, who are kept en masse in "battery cages", stacked on top of each other inside of large warehouse-type facilities. In fact, most hens *and* chickens spend their entire lives in wire crates, packed so tightly that it's impossible for them to spread their wings. Out of frustration and fear they often peck at each other and are sometimes found dead or wounded.

All factory farm animals are run through an assembly-line system of slaughter due to the volume of supply needed to keep up with demand.

More than 150 billion animals are killed each year for human consumption[2,3]. That's BILLION with a B! Out of that 150 billion an estimated 70 to 80 billion are land animals. This means that approximately 219 million land animals are killed each day of every year. Broken down even further, this equates to over 9 million per hour, more than 152,000 killed every minute, or nearly 2,600 slaughtered every single second of every single day! Put another way, in the time it takes you to blink, more than 2,500 land animals lose their lives.

At this non-stop pace it's easy to understand why animals are frequently still wide awake when the fur is boiled off their bodies and they are skinned or butchered while still aware and able to feel pain. In fact, some factory farm workers have complained that it's nearly impossible to render an animal completely unconscious, as is legally required, in the short period of time they have to load their bodies onto conveyor belts. CAFO workers also point out that the accelerated processing speed does not allow for proper inspection of the carcasses, making it possible for tainted meat to go unnoticed before being packaged and sold to consumers[4,5].

In addition to the processing mistakes that take place on factory farms, there's an unfathomable amount of physical, and sometimes even sexual abuse, to which these helpless animals are subjected on a regular basis[4,6-7]. Yet, when safety inspectors object and attempt to voice concerns they're frequently told to ignore the infractions or specifically instructed to *not* file formal reports. Rather than protecting the animals and the consumers who pay their salaries, some officials choose to protect factory farm owners and their employees instead. High level regulators have gone as far as taking action against federal inspectors who report the violations. One such federal meat inspector and veterinarian, Dean Wyatt, testified in a congressional hearing in 2010[7]. In his testimony he stated that his authority was constantly undermined and that he was frequently mocked by factory farm workers and plant managers. Wyatt condemned the system and his superiors, stating that he was often the victim of harassment and intimidation, having had his job threatened numerous times, experiencing verbal admonitions and assaults regularly, and being demoted at one point, all for doing his job to the best of his ability.

> *"If factory farms had glass walls,*
> *everyone would be vegetarian"*
>
> ~Paul McCartney

Wyatt also affirmed that reports had been deleted and that the verbiage in some documents had been modified, in an effort to cover up abusive behaviors. An example he provided involved a male calf, only days old, who had been violently thrown "off the second tier of the hauling trailer like a football" because the calf was too weak from several days drive without food or water, to lift himself and walk. However, after filing an official report regarding the incident, it was altered and the word "dropped" was substituted for the word "threw".

Wyatt's testimony contained numerous, additional accounts of direct violations of the Humane Methods of Slaughter Act and the Federal Meat Inspection Act. He provided details stating that pigs were often conscious when their throats were slit and animals were regularly handled in an abusive manner with some being hit, yelled at, and/or dragged about. Wyatt went on to recount his experience at a New England CAFO, where rifles are used to shoot cattle with a bullet as a means of "stunning" the animal. He testified that, "a cow was shot once near her eye, again in her nose, and was still standing, fully conscious, and obviously suffering."

A tremendous amount of physical pain is also inflicted through standard farming practices. Some of these "standard practices" include dehorning, castration, tail- docking, beak removal, and branding. In producers' efforts to boost profits and keep the production line moving quickly, the animals are made to endure these excruciating procedures without pain medication of any kind.

Another agonizing practice is the use of a hose forced down a calf's esophagus to relieve pressure caused by the unnatural diet on factory farms[8]. A cow's natural diet consists of grass. However, to speed up the growth process and increase profitability, factory farmers strictly feed calves corn and soy grain after only a few months of life and up until slaughter. The unnatural diet can negatively react with a calf's ruminant system, especially when the change is made too quickly. This causes their rumen, one of a cow's 2 stomachs, to fill with gas and exert pressure on the lungs, resulting in suffocation if the condition is not relieved with a hose. In addition to the feedlot bloat, as it's called on factory farms, the consumption of corn changes the pH level in a cow's stomach, making it highly acidic. Consequently, the animal experiences a great deal of pain and discomfort. According to Michael Pollen, author of *In Defense of Food*, this abnormally high state of acidity can result in diarrhea, ulcers, liver disease, and a weakened immune system[9].

While some might like to think that the most vile and deplorable acts of cruelty on factory farms–the intentional physical and sexual abuse–are isolated incidents, and that they happen only on rare occasions, I promise you that such is not the case. Time and again undercover investigators have witnessed, documented, and filmed horrific cases of cruelty, and it has been going on for decades, even in so-called "humane" meat production facilities[10,11]. It is only now, due largely to the Internet and technological advances in recording devices, that we're learning about the depravity and sadistic behavior of factory farm workers.

As the cases mount, the meat industry has taken steps to silence and ban animal-welfare investigators by lobbying government officials to introduce what is known as "ag gag" legislation[12]. These laws, if enacted, make it illegal for investigators to record what happens in and on the farms. The laws go so far as to criminalize undercover investigators, granting factory farm owners the ability to press charges and potentially prosecute the very people attempting to protect animals from abuse and negligence. The blatant and sole purpose of these proposed laws is to keep the public in the dark regarding what goes on inside factory farms and to protect the meat and dairy industries. But in the words of Dr. Phil McGraw, "He who has nothing to hide hides nothing."

Why or how could someone willfully stab, beat, stomp, kick, or even sexually assault an animal? Many people have theories, including the fact that some factory farm workers have criminal records, so they're prone to violence in the only job they can get. Others speculate that factory farm laborers are simply taking out their frustration on the animals because of the exhausting pace at which they're forced to move the animals through the process. Some even believe that the process itself, of routine killing, is enough to send anyone "over the edge" and that workers in the industry have to desensitize themselves to suffering in order to get through the day. There is some evidence to support this theory. I have been told that Foster Farms provides free psychiatric care for their employees to help them cope with what they witness and experience on the job.

Although there's truth in all of these theories, I believe that to even consider such a job a person would have to be lacking in empathy. I question who could stand by and watch, day in and day out, as animals fought for their lives and as the life drained from their eyes.

I don't believe that anyone with the least degree of compassion could witness and be unaffected by the incomprehensible suffering that occurs on factory farms. Even on dairy farms where animals are not killed, workers witness a calf, fresh out of its mother's womb, being literally dragged away as both mother and baby bellow in grief. It is reported that mother cows bellow for so long and so hard that their throats are left raw after several weeks of non-stop crying. There even have been accounts of cows that have hidden their calves in an effort to keep them from being taken away. Clearly they feel the grief of losing their offspring, just as a human being would.

Can you imagine how much harder a mother cow would bellow if she knew the truth about what awaited her calf on a factory farm.

When a male calf is born, he is subjected to the excruciating pain of dehorning, castration, branding, and possibly tail-docking, all without the use of sedatives or pain killers. When he reaches maturity, typically before the age of three years old, he'll be killed for his meat and/or his hide. If he's one of the truly unlucky males, he'll be confined to a windowless crate, so small that he cannot stand up or turn around. He'll spend four solid months alone in that dark box, lying in his own feces and urine, until he is dragged off to the slaughterhouse floor, to be cut into veal steaks.

If the mother cow gives birth to a female, the calf will most likely be taken to a dairy farm where she'll be forcefully impregnated by use of the "rape rack," a device that holds the female calf in place while she is inseminated. Like her mother, she'll spend her entire life giving birth, over and over again, only to experience the loss of her own calf after each pregnancy. At the age of only four to five years old she too will be taken to a slaughterhouse and rewarded for her dairy production by being hung upside down by her hind legs. Just as the males experience at the slaughterhouse, her hips will pop out of joint and her ligaments will rip apart as she thrashes and fights for her life, causing the most horrific pain. Her throat will then be slit, and she'll move along the conveyor belt. One can only hope that she will bleed out and become unconscious before she is skinned to make leather or her limbs are severed and she is cut into steaks and roasts. Sadly, as we now know, this is rarely the case.

Chickens fare no better than cows when it comes to standard slaughter methods. To maintain a rigorous pace there are typically two ways in which chickens, hens, turkeys and all other winged animals are killed. All are hung by their legs and move along a conveyor belt upside down, but the mode of slaughter varies from farm to farm. Some farms use a blade to slice the throat of the animal as it moves, thereby bleeding the animal to death. Others employ electrocution, wherein the animal has their head submerged into water charged with electricity.

Even the egg industry is fraught with inhumane practices that horrify any rational human being. Take, for instance, the treatment of male chicks. They are, for the most part, useless in this segment of the industry. Therefore, they are either left to suffocate in garbage bags, along with hundreds of other males, or fed directly into a meat grinder while still alive. Often these ground-up chicks are used as feed for the egg-laying hens.

The feeding of dead animals to the same species is not an anomaly in factory farming, as the industry is well known for cannibalizing animals raised for human consumption. In fact, "downer" animals–those too ill to be raised to full size or sold as meat–are frequently slaughtered and used to feed healthy animals on factory farms. Obviously this practice poses its own set of problems since there is no way to determine whether these sick animals were suffering from a disease that could be passed on to the animals that humans consume.

The cannibalization of sick animals may be a moot issue, however, since there have been cases involving the sale of meat from downer cows directly to consumers. In 2007 the Westland/Hallmark Meat Company, based in Chino Hills, California, was the subject of an undercover investigation which revealed not only deplorable animal abuse, but the slaughter and sale of sick cows[13]. This investigation led to the largest beef recall in history. The company admitted, however, after being caught, that the majority of the tainted beef had most likely been consumed prior to the recall. To make matters worse, this company was a supplier for school lunch programs.

Knowing all this, it is difficult to believe that any compassionate, non-sadistic human being would *choose* this kind of job, and then *stay* in it. So then, by the very nature of the work itself, only those with little to no regard for life would be attracted to such work. Therefore, abuse, neglect, and cruelty are inevitable so long as there is a market for animal products.

7

I'd Rather Go Blind

The image that has stuck with me the longest is a picture of a pig desperately clawing at the sides of a large vat of boiling water. The caption under the photo explained that, although pigs are suppose to be stunned with a gun before being strung up by their hind legs and carried along the processing line, many awaken due to improper stunning procedures. The pig I saw was wide awake when she was dropped into the boiling water to remove the hair from her body. Her attempts to escape the unimaginable pain were futile, and she died in agony.

This image, more than many others, is seared into my memory because it was nearly identical to a photo taken at a dog-meat market in Thailand that I had seen just one year earlier. The photo of the small dog was heart-wrenching. She too was clawing at the side of a pot as the water's temperature continued to rise. According to animal activists who posted the photo, she tried desperately to escape, but her fate was sealed.

It was this photo of the wet, tea-cup-sized dog, along with several others, that fired me up and turned me into an activist against the trade in dog and cat meat in Southeast Asia.

If you've never heard of this vile animal meat trade, you're not alone. Many people are completely unaware of the fact that every year approximately seven million dogs and hundreds of thousands of cats are tortured, then skinned or boiled alive and eaten in Southeast Asian countries. This practice isn't because the people in those countries are starving and have no other choice. To many in this part of the world, dog meat is actually considered to be a delicacy and can cost as much as four times the price of beef. In addition, it is a cultural belief that the more an animal suffers before it dies, the more health benefits its meat will have. This is why it is standard practice to string up large dogs by their necks and place small dogs and cats in bags, to beat them with rods or sticks, before boiling or skinning them. Many of these animals are pets stolen from loving homes, while others are strays or born and raised in dog-meat farms for the sole purpose of being eaten.

As soon as I learned about this barbaric practice, I knew that I had to take action. I wasted no time, and along with my daughter and a good friend I went door to door and stood outside our local grocery store handing out flyers.

A year later, as I sat looking at the picture of the pig in that large vat of boiling hot water, tears welled up in my eyes, and the realization dawned that I had been a complete hypocrite. I wept. Not streaming tears but deep, gut-wrenching sobs of pain for all the living creatures that had been abused, tortured, and killed for the sake of my taste buds.

I considered what this was costing me. What was the true cost to my soul if I did nothing or if I changed nothing?

What was the price of silence and inaction?

World-famous women's rights activist Zainab Salbi has said that when we choose to look the other way when we see injustice, "we allow for the corruption of our own values."

I agree, and I now recognize that when we choose to ignore the suffering of others, even if it's "only an animal," the consequences are immense. Indifference to suffering is like a poison that seeps into every crack and crevice of our lives. It stains the moral fiber of our being and permeates and makes toxic the marrow of our soul. Like a cancer caused by that toxicity, we can remove a section of the disease, but another mass will surely surface somewhere else unless and until we heal the root cause–our lack of empathy. To do this, we must excise our apathy tumor and correct the stigmatisms of our heart that prevents us from taking action against that which we know is wrong, and from truly seeing what we deem unpleasant or disturbing.

I believe that if we take no action and make no effort to right the wrong, choosing instead to deny the reality and the consequences of our habits, we become severed from the essence of our being–the soul that longs to carry out its divinely appointed mission of unselfish love here on Earth.

> *"The time will come when men*
> *such as I will look upon the murder of animals*
> *as now they look upon the murder of men"*
>
> ~Leonardo da Vinci

8

All My Fault

Over the coming months, as I came to understand that the botched, painful deaths and abuse of animals were not uncommon, I began to question how and why these practices were allowed to continue. What I discovered is that there are four reasons: politics, greed, you, and I.

Right about now you might be saying, "Whatchyou talkin' 'bout Willis/Gina? I would never endorse violence against animals or willingly accept painful and cruel slaughter practices."

While I understand your sentiments, and I was once right there with you, we are complicit every day that we *choose* to put animal products on our plate and into our bodies.

In her popular TEDx talk titled "Beyond Carnism," Harvard-trained psychologist Melanie Joy offers an explanation for how otherwise intelligent and compassionate human beings rationalize the killing and consumption of other living creatures[1]. She states that we "distort our thoughts, numb our feelings, and act against our core values."

Dr. Joy goes on to say that of approximately seven million species on the planet, people tend to regard only a handful as edible.

Think about that for a moment and ask yourself this question: Why do you eat only certain animals? Do you have a logical answer, or is it a case of just what you were taught was "normal" and acceptable?

When I look back, I can't believe that I never addressed this question. I remember a conversation with my husband years ago that demonstrates our complacency and "blindness" when it comes to a traditionally accepted practice. We were talking about a lady we both knew who had a large piece of property in a neighboring city and was raising about a half dozen pot-belly pigs that she had rescued. Given her proclivity for rescuing pigs, I asked him whether she ate pork or not. He replied, "Probably. Those are different kinds of pigs than the ones she rescues." At the time it made perfect sense to me, and I never gave it a second thought, but now it just seems insane. I mean, who made these rules? Who decided that one type of animal, or in this anecdote one type of pig, is okay for humans to eat while others aren't?

Eating only certain animals is a learned behavior, and it varies depending on what country you live in. Here in America we are repulsed by the idea of eating a dog or cat, and we think that people in Southeast Asia must be sociopaths for doing so. However, in India people believe that cows are sacred, and I'm sure they regard the rest of the world as disgusting and sacrilegious for consuming beef. Then there's Muslims, who believe that pigs are unclean. I would imagine that they're horrified by the Western obsession with bacon and other pork products on and in every meal.

Like me, you probably never made a connection between that slab of brownish, reddish meat sitting on your plate and the playful, affectionate cow who had a beating heart and a desire to live, just as your dog or cat. You probably also never imagined that these animals were being abused or killed in a gruesome manner, or that dairy cows suffer for years before slaughter, having their newborn babies ripped away just minutes after giving birth. I know that I didn't, but I also admit that I never took the time to learn about what was really happening. I assumed (and you know what assume stands for–making an "ass" out of "u" and "me") that if it were wrong someone would stop it. Then I realized that I'm someone. We're all that "someone." I was then faced with the question of, as "someone", what am *I* going to do about it?

I understood, for the first time in my life, that it was *my* responsibility as a human being to require more of myself. It no longer made sense to eat another living creature. The thought of preparing and biting into a farm animal's flesh became as repulsive to me as biting into one of my dogs, whom I consider to be family. The path, however, remained a bit hazy. I still wasn't sure how I would put the whole plant-based diet thing into practice, but now I had the determination and will to figure it out. And, as they say, where there's a will there's a way. When I'm determined to do something, I have the will of ten sumo wrestlers, so it's best to lower your safety bar, keep your arms and legs inside the ride and hold on tight.

My husband and daughter were in for a surprise.

9

World Destruction

After studying vast amounts of scientific research, and in my formal training, I've come to understand that eating animals is not only unnecessary but also extremely unhealthy, even toxic, for humans.

Animals raised on factory farms are the most lethal of all. As mentioned, large profits are the primary objective in factory farming, which is why animals are fed growth hormones to make them grow abnormally large within a short period of time.

Drugs prohibited for use in humans are routinely fed as additives to livestock to increase the yield of meat and maximize profits. One such drug, ractopamine[1,2], reduces the amount of fat on an animal while increasing the proportion of lean meat. This drug is used in the raising of pigs, cows, and turkey and is in a class known as beta-adrenergic agonists. It mimics stress hormones in the animal's body, such as epinephrine and norepinephrine, making the heart beat faster and causing the heart muscle to contract. It's also believed to make the animals more vulnerable to heat.

While ractopamine is banned from use in food production in approximately 160 countries, it has yet to be eliminated in animal production in the United States. As is all too common in the U.S., the FDA initially relied on studies performed by the drug maker in determining the safety of ractopamine for farm animals. Those studies focused primarily on the cost-effective nature of various doses in relation to rate of growth. Conspicuously absent from the research were any data pertaining to animal welfare or the drug's effect on human health. This is especially concerning due to the fact that in independent animal research and studies, ractopamine has been shown to cause reproductive dysfunction, birth defects, disability, and early death. In humans, ractopamine is known to disturb the cardiovascular system and can trigger hyperactivity, elevated heart rates, and palpitations. Evidence also suggests that it causes chromosomal abnormalities and behavioral changes, and the Pork Trade Chamber of Commerce in China reports that over a 12-year period, 1,700 people were poisoned as a result of consuming ractopamine-tainted pork. Possibly even more alarming is a ractopamine drug label, which provides evidence of its danger to humans and should make everyone reconsider their menu for Thanksgiving dinner. Topmax, the version of ractopamine used in turkey feed, contains the following text[2]:

"WARNING: The active ingredient in Topmax, ractopamine hydrochloride, is a beta-adrenergic agonist. Individuals with cardiovascular disease should exercise special caution to avoid exposure. Not for use in humans. Keep out of the reach of children. The Topmax 9 formulation (Type A Medicated Article) poses a low dust potential under usual conditions of handling and mixing. When mixing and handling Topmax, use protective clothing, impervious gloves, protective eye wear, and a NIOSH-approved dust mask. Operators should wash thoroughly with soap and water after handling. If accidental eye contact occurs, immediately rinse eyes thoroughly with water. If irritation persists, seek medical attention."

Another beta-adrenergic agonist used in factory farming is zilpaterol, more commonly referred to by its commercial name, Zilmax. The use of this weight-promoting drug is more disturbing because it is said to be 125 times more potent than ractopamine. Unlike ractopamine, Zilmax is actually approved for human consumption and the FDA has shown little interest in the drug's potentially harmful effects on humans, even though it has proven deadly for cows[3] and has been shown to cause tachycardia, muscle tremors, and renal damage in horses[4].

Zilmax is believed to be responsible for hoof loss, with farmers reporting that their cow's hooves have just fallen off. Animal experts say that this is as painful as "walking on glass" and, as a result, the animals are euthanized. The FDA's own reports attribute stomach ulcers, brain lesions, and blindness in cattle to the drug's use, and the manufacturer of the drug, Merck, noted lethargy, bloody noses, respiratory issue, and heart failure in animals that had been fed Zilmax. Factory farm owners have also reported an increase in mortality rates and feedlot bloat while using the drug, and data collected by the USDA show that euthanization figures surged after the weight promoter was introduced in the U.S. In fact, euthanization rates rose 175% in the two-year period after Zilmax sales began. This drug, like many others fed to animals raised for human consumption, has been found in the urine, plasma, muscle, and internal organs of slaughtered animals[5,6].

In addition to ractopamine, Zilmax, and similar drugs, factory farm animals are pumped full of antibiotics. Like ractopamine, some act as growth hormones, making the animals grow larger, in a condensed time period. Others are used to counter the poor conditions and unethical manner in which the animals are raised. Because space is limited, animals are crammed together living on and in their own waste, as well as that of their fellow farm mates. However, these unsanitary conditions cause disease and illness in the herds. To combat these issues, and as a matter of standard practice, farmers began injecting their livestock with a staggering amount of antibiotics, so much so that a reported 70–80% of all antibiotics sold in the United States[7] and approximately 50% of antibiotics sold in the United Kingdom[29] are used for factory farm animals. These drugs are then stored in the animals' tissue and organs and passed on to the humans who consume them. Excess antibiotics are excreted via urine and feces and often find their way into our drinking water. In addition, factory farm manure is often used to fertilize plant crops that humans and animals eat on a daily basis.

The use of antibiotics in livestock production is of major concern for several reasons. The first is that humans are becoming antibiotic resistant[8,9]. As in the preantibiotic era, people are dying from basic illnesses and diseases that should be easily cured. In years past these ailments would have responded to treatment with routine antibiotics. However, because of their daily ingestion of such drugs, most people have developed an immunity to them. Considering that farmers have even been caught giving numerous antibiotics to dairy cows, which is strictly prohibited unless a cow is ill, it's easy to understand how this situation has become a serious matter[10]. Deaths have even been reported in adults and children who were suffering from simple bacteria-related illnesses. Normally these patients would have responded to a course of antibiotic treatment.

Instead, they died from diarrhea-induced dehydration as a result of antibiotic resistance. This debility has become so common that, according to the CDC, 23,000 Americans die annually due to "super-bug" infections[8].

The overuse of antibiotics gained a great deal of national attention in 2015 when the UK Prime Minister commissioned a report titled *Antimicrobials in Agriculture and the Environment: Reducing Unnecessary Use and Waste,* by an international advisory group[11]. The report stated that, unless swift, corrective action is taken, drug-resistant strains of tuberculosis, malaria, HIV, and certain bacterial infections could cause the deaths of 10 million people annually by the year 2050.

Another danger of antibiotic consumption is the damage it does to our immune system, leaving us even more vulnerable to infections, illnesses, diseases, and disorders. Approximately 70% of our immune system resides in our gut lining and the "community" of good and bad bacteria in our body known as our microbiome. Proper balance of our gut bacteria, also called our gut flora, is essential because this is our first line of defense against any illness or disease, including cancer.

Maintaining healthy gut bacteria can protect you against diabetes, atherosclerosis, autoimmune diseases, inflammatory bowel disease, liver disease, diarrhea, asthma, and hormonal imbalances[12]. In addition to disturbing the balance of bacteria in your gut, some antibiotics have been shown to produce inflammation in the intestinal lining and reduce the viscosity of beneficial mucus in the intestines[13]. This can lead to or exacerbate a painful condition called colitis, and can compromise the gut lining, making it possible for foreign substances to enter your blood stream, causing an autoimmune response.

Good bacteria help to regulate your metabolism, keeping you fit and lean, and an imbalance between good and bad gut flora, or a decrease in microbial diversity, has been directly linked to obesity[12,14]. Several studies and reports show the connection between gut bacteria and obesity. An animal study[15] published in 2015 established a direct correlation between early antibiotic consumption and increased bone and body mass due to changes in the microbiome. The study further revealed that the effects of some antibiotics are long lasting, with scientists noting abnormal biological functions and disruption of metabolism in test subjects. These findings indicate that antibiotics consumed, even early in life, can lead to weight management issues as an adult. An earlier report from 2010 detailed the effects of gut bacteria imbalance on metabolic inflammation within the body[16]. Scientists explained that the imbalance and inflammation ultimately results in insulin resistance and obesity. While fiber-rich plant foods are miraculous in helping to support, rebuild, and strengthen our colonies of good gut bacteria, antibiotics are like a wrecking ball that destroys everything in its path, leaving our bodies with little to no immune defense.

As you can imagine, animals raised for food are also developing a resistance to antibiotics, resulting recently in the deaths of 10% of the pig population in the United States. In 2014 a virus known as Porcine Epidemic Diarrhea (PEDv) swept through the U.S. and spread to parts of Canada and Mexico, killing huge numbers of pigs, and causing the price of pork to soar[17]. At one time, PEDv was easily treated with antibiotics. However, it has now become nearly 100% fatal due to antibiotic resistance in farm animals. To combat this deadly virus, farmers are feeding the intestines, carcasses, and manure from the dead, infected pigs, to the still healthy pigs or spraying a mixture of water and contaminated manure into the healthy pigs' nostrils[18]. When this is done, the healthy pigs supposedly become ill for a few days as they develop a natural immunity to the PED virus. They also pass the immunity onto their piglets. These exposed and "immune" pigs are then slaughtered and sold for human consumption.

The widespread issue of antibiotic resistance revealed itself again in 2015 when tests performed in China revealed that pigs infected with E.coli had built up a resistance to Colistin by way of a specific gene, MCR-1[19,20]. This antibiotic-resistant gene appeared in 21% of the animals tested and 15% of raw meat samples, between 2008 and 2013. Scientists say that the prevalence of MCR-1 increased year over year, indicating that the gene is spreading. Pigs with positive results were immune to even "last-defense" drugs such as Colistin because of its overuse in animal agriculture. Upon further investigation, researchers realized that this MCR-1 gene, and subsequent immunity, could actually transfer to other strains of bacteria, something that had never occurred before. Simply put, any MCR-1 gene-carrying being is at risk of death should they contract *any* type of bacterial infection because antibiotics would be useless. What made this discovery even more terrifying is that scientists found the same MCR-1 gene in 16 patients, admitted to the hospital for infection. It was also later found in a Danish patient and poultry samples in Denmark, indicating that MCR-1 has the ability to cross from one species to another. Clearly, this gene poses a serious threat to the survival of all life. Scientists are calling for the cessation of Colistin and other similar last-defense antibiotics in factory farming, as they believe that this is the "start of the antibiotic apocalypse."[21]

What about the PED virus previously mentioned? Can it be transferred to humans? Scientists say no, but they've been wrong before. The Bovine Leukemia Virus (BLV) causes cancer in approximately 5% of infected animals, most specifically malignant lymphoma and lymphosarcoma. Although a

2007 USDA survey revealed that 100% of the cows on large dairy farms (those with 500+ cows) tested positive for BLV, consumers were assured that this virus could not be transmitted to humans[22]. Government officials also claimed that, even if BLV could be transferred, it was harmless to humans, so there was nothing to worry about. However, a 2014 study conducted by University of California at Berkeley scientists proved otherwise when they found BLV in human breast tissue. Upon further investigation scientists discovered that BLV is not only present but also prevalent in the breast tissue of women with breast cancer. Their 2015 study revealed that 59% of the cancer samples tested contained BLV, which comes from cow's milk and the blood cells and mammary tissue of cattle[23,24]. The findings indicate that the presence of BLV places women at greater risk for breast cancer than obesity, alcohol consumption, or even synthetic hormone replacement therapy, all of which were previously considered to be the highest risk factors of all.

Although BLV is pervasive throughout the U.S., the virus is not exclusive to the western world. Other countries have begun testing for BLV and have found that the virus is not as common, but does exist. Of 1,116 herds tested in Turkey[25], 11.82% were found to house animals infected with BLV. Likewise, a study conducted in Iran[26] testing cows, sheep, and camels revealed that camels appear to be immune to BLV. However, of the 874 blood samples collected, 17.2%

of the cattle and sheep tested positive. Similar tests have been performed in Peru, Paraguay, and Bolivia[27], with up to 50% of cows testing positive for the virus. Given that BLV is transferred by blood, it can easily be spread to other members of the herd via tools used in standard farming practices (e.g.: dehorning, tail-docking, castration, injections) and to newborn calves from infected mothers, or calves that are fed from tanks containing milk from numerous cows[28].

Another potentially deadly medical condition now associated with animals and the overuse of antibiotics[29] is Methicillin-resistant Staphylococcus aureus (MRSA). MRSA is known to cause skin and soft tissue infections that can lead to death, in severe cases. This antibiotic-resistant infection has now morphed into what is called Livestock Associated Methicillin-resistant Staphylcoccus aureus (LA-MRSA or MRSA CC398), and it can even be transferred to newborn humans through the mother's umbilical cord. LA-MRSA can be contracted in several ways, including handling of raw meat or physical contact with an infected animal or human carrier. In addition, U.S. studies have shown that those living within close proximity to factory farms, or near fields where manure is sprayed, are at greater risk of becoming infected with this dangerous bacterial infection[30].

Although LA-MRSA is most commonly found in factory-farmed pigs, it has also been identified in cows, chickens, and dogs, and the bacteria has been discovered in pork, chicken, and turkey products in the U.S. What's truly disturbing is that many countries, including the UK, do not even test for this strain of MRSA, and it is reported that approximately 60–70% of Danish pig farmers are carriers of the bacterium. In addition, 70% of the farms sampled in Denmark tested positive for LA-MRSA. There have also been reported cases of infected humans in the United States and Canada.

While overuse of antibiotics may be a driving factor in the proliferation of LA-MRSA and the difficulty found in treating such infections, scientists warn that farm animals raised without the use of antibiotics still test positive for strains of MRSA bacteria[31].

Now let's talk about arsenic. Not something you think of immediately, when you're talking about animal foods, I know. Nevertheless, arsenic, which is a known carcinogen[32] and is associated with an increased risk of cancer, diabetes, neurological disorders, and cardiovascular disease[33,35], has been used in animal production for decades, especially on U.S. factory farms that produce chicken.

According to the USDA, there are 430 parts per billion of arsenic in one serving of chicken. They also state that chickens produced in the United States consume two million pounds of chemicals containing arsenic annually[34], and the U.S. Department of Health and Human Services attributes 80% of arsenic intake by humans to contaminated meat, fish, and poultry[35]. In a 2004 USDA research article[36], scientists stated that the mean concentration of total arsenic in young chickens was three to four times higher than what's found in other poultry and meat.

So what is the arsenic used for? Well, even though the use of this toxic substance was banned in Europe more than a decade ago, U.S. meat producers received approval from the FDA to use arsenic in animal feed to kill internal parasites, increase weight, and "improve pigmentation" in pigs, chickens, and turkey. This was after they determined that consumers prefer to purchase animal meat with a pink hue.

Considering that we already have a certain level of arsenic circulating as a natural element in our bodies, we can easily exceed safe levels. In addition to the arsenic found in animal meat, our bodies absorb this toxic substance from other foods[37] and environmental pollutants. Arsenic also has the ability to cross the placenta, making it a danger to unborn babies[35]. It's also important to note that consumption of chicken has increased substantially over the years. A *Huffington Post* article in January, 2014, cited USDA statistics[38] reflecting that, for the first time in history, Americans were eating more chicken than beef. I concluded two things from this article: (1) those Chick-fil-A signs are working; and (2) consumers are completely unaware that they have a toxic piece of animal flesh sitting on their plate.

In 2013, the FDA agreed to withdraw the approval of *some* arsenic drugs used in animal agriculture[39]. The about face was in response to public pressure following a 2013 Johns Hopkin's study and a lawsuit filed by consumer advocacy group, Center for Food Safety[40,41]. The lawsuit was based on the findings of the study, which proved that organic arsenic, used in animal feed, converts to the cancer-causing, inorganic version of arsenic after consumption. The advocacy group later filed another complaint against the FDA alleging that the government agency was attempting to conceal documents pertaining to the safety of arsenic, after they failed to comply with a Freedom of Information Act (FOIA) request for arsenic-related studies and copies of communications with arsenic drug manufacturers[42]. Finally in 2015, the FDA announced that it would withdraw approval of the final arsenic-based drug used in animal feed[43]. While this is great news, it does not mean that farmers will comply or that they won't substitute another, equally dangerous drug for arsenic, as they try to find a way to escape the consequences of raising tens of thousands of animals in cramped and unsanitary living conditions. Based on historical evidence, we can be certain that farmers will use another inexpensive and potentially toxic substance to control the inevitable diseases and illnesses, or the cost to manufacture chicken, turkey, and pork products will increase considerably.

Clearly there are a lot of "added ingredients" in animal products that most people are not aware of, and we're just now realizing that these substances have a detrimental effect on our well-being, in spite of government and food industry reassurances.

One of the things that make us susceptible to overconsumption of dangerous substances is flawed scientific recommendations based on archaic methods used by government agencies to determine a level of safety. For instance, the FDA often determines that a particular food is acceptable for human consumption because the amount of drugs or toxins it contains is within safe levels. However, regulatory agencies consider only one source of exposure when making these determinations. While those methods of testing may have worked at one time in history, you and I are now being assaulted by toxins, drugs, and chemicals day and night, leaving us vulnerable to overexposure or unforeseen interactions among them.

10

Weird Science

As if immune-system damage and being poisoned weren't enough, you now have to contend with the DNA damage and gut lining destruction caused by genetically modified organisms, otherwise known as GMOs. But what are GMOs, and why are they so devastating to our bodies?

Although genetic modification, also called genetic engineering or gene splicing, has been used in numerous ways for centuries, scientists have taken this practice to an entirely new level by developing two types of dangerous seeds. These are herbicide-resistant seeds and BT seeds, and they pose one of the biggest threats to human health today[1-3].

GMO seeds, which now are used to grow 85–90% of crops in the United States and approximately 30–80% of the crops throughout the world, are created by genetically altering plant species at the DNA level. In this case, the "engineered plants have been merged with bacteria, viruses, animals, and other plants to make crops resistant to drought, herbicides, pesticides, and infestation and to increase yield. Unfortunately, none of these objectives were achieved, and even worse we now know that pesticide and herbicide use has actually *increased* with the proliferation of herbicide-resistant GMO crops, also known as Roundup Ready crops. It consequently has become necessary to develop even stronger herbicides and pesticides, as weeds have evolved and are now resistant[4-6] to Roundup and similar products, becoming what are known as "super weeds."

Roundup in particular has proven to be extremely hazardous to human health. The International Agency for Research on Cancer (IARC), a department of the World Health Organization (WHO), evaluated glyphosate, the key ingredient in Roundup, and classified it as a Level 2A Carcinogen[7].

The WHO is responsible for researching and vetting *all* available scientific literature and disseminating scientific facts as they relate to the health of human beings throughout the world. WHO reports are considered to be the "gold standard" and their findings are above reproach because this preeminent, international organization is not influenced by special-interest groups.

The IARC's classification means that they have identified

glyphosate as "probably carcinogenic to humans." Their report further states that there is "sufficient evidence of carcinogenicity in experimental animals" and that "glyphosate also caused DNA and chromosomal damage in human cells." Additional studies show a connection between glyphosate consumption and a host of neurological disorders, including depression, dementia, autism, anxiety disorder, and Parkinson's disease[8].

In addition to multiple types of cancer, glyphosate has been linked either directly or indirectly to the following health conditions and concerns[9-15,38]:

ADHD

Antibiotic resistance

Birth defects

Brain fog

Cataracts

Crohn's disease

Congenital head and facial malformations

Congenital urogenital malformations

Down's syndrome

Endocrine disruption

Eye disorders

Fetal malnutrition

Heart disorders

Hepatitis

Immune system disorders

Increased estrogen in men

Increased testosterone in women

Infertility

Inflammatory bowel disease

Kidney damage

Liver disease

Lung disorders

Lymphatic disorders

Magnesium deficiency

Malformations of heart and lungs

Miscarriage

Mitochondrial dysfunction

Organ damage

Oxidative damage

Respiratory issues

Skin disorders

Slow fetal growth

Spontaneous abortion

Still births

Thymus malformation

Thyroid disorders

Tumor formation

When tested as an individual substance, glyphosate causes human cells to die just as Roundup does. Other ingredients, adjuvants in Roundup, are said to be "inert". However, they've been proven to magnify the damaging effects of glyphosate and, when mixed, are far more toxic, even at levels well below the FDAs approved limit[16]. Studies show that, when combined, the solvents contained in the Roundup herbicide increase the permeability of your mitochondrial membranes, making it easier for glyphosate to enter. In addition, both Roundup and individual, various adjuvants found in the formula damage cell membranes and poison your mitochondria. Testing on glyphosate alone showed that it too poisons the mitochondria, but without damaging the cell membrane[17,18].

This explains the almost epidemic level of chronic fatigue and disease rates we're witnessing throughout the world because your mitochondria are akin to little energy producing factories and there are hundreds to thousands within each cell of your body. They're also instrumental in controlling inflammation[19] and promoting apoptosis[20], the automatic self-destruction of damaged cells. This process occurs naturally in the human body to prevent abnormal cells from reproducing uncontrollably and becoming a tumor. Subsequently, when your mitochondria are damaged, you are at greater risk for developing cancer.

Mitochondrial damage is also believed to cause cancer due to the resulting change in energy production within the cell, from aerobic (seen in cells with abundant and healthy mitochondria) to aerobic glycolysis or anaerobic (seen in cells with damaged and fewer mitochondria). When a cell generates energy via glycolysis (via the breakdown of glucose), it produces a potentially toxic substance called lactic acid. Nobel prize winner, Dr. Otto Warburg, asserted and scientifically substantiated that this shift to glycolysis and the resulting lactic acid was responsible for the development of cancer cells[22,23]. In addition to cancer, mitochondria dysfunction is related to and involved in the following diseases and disorders[23-29]:

Abdominal pain

Allergies

ALS

Alzheimer's disease

Asthma

Atherosclerosis

Autism

Autoimmune disease

Bi-polar disorder

Chronic fatigue syndrome

Constipation

Depression

Diarrhea

Epilepsy

Fibromyalgia

Heart disease

High blood pressure

Huntington's disease

Hypertension

Hypotonia

Metabolic syndrome

Migraines

Neuropathy

Obesity

Parkinson's disease

Schizophrenia

Seizure disorders

Type 2 diabetes

The second genetically modified seed known as BT *(Bacillus thuringiensis)* may even be worse than the kind from which Roundup Ready crops are grown because it is engineered with a form of bacterium that produces a toxic protein. Therefore, there's no need to spray pesticides or herbicides on these plants, because the toxin resides within every cell of the plant itself. Consequently, when an insect bites into the plant, it ingests the toxin, which breaks the insect's stomach apart, killing it instantly. Yet the makers of BT seeds claim that this edible explosive is harmless to humans because it's excreted before it can do any damage or before it can be stored in the body. However, a 2011 study[30] conducted in Canada revealed that this toxin is not only stored in the body, but passed on to newborn babies. Scientists found BT toxin in the umbilical cord of 93% of the pregnant women tested, and in 80% of umbilical blood tested. In nonpregnant women the BT toxin was present in 67% of study participants.

Of grave concern, biologist and former GMO scientist, Jonathan Latham points out that the BT toxin is "indistinguishable from the well-known anthrax bacterium" and it shares "structural similarities" with the lethal poison, ricin[31].

Several scientists have raised concerns regarding genetically engineered plants containing a viral gene known as gene VI[32-34]. This gene comes from the Cauliflower Mosaic Virus

(CaMV) and its purpose is to weaken resistance to specific pathogens by disrupting the immune process that normally provides protection in plants[34]. The question is, what then, does gene VI do to the human immune system? Unfortunately there is no answer to that question because no testing has been performed to assess the risk of gene VI[33-35], so it could have far-reaching and dangerous effects with long-term consumption. Government regulatory agencies and the scientific community have absolutely no way of knowing, yet this gene can be found in more than half of the genetically modified plants approved for human and animal consumption in the United States. What is known is that the virus was found in the blood, liver, and brain tissue of experimental rats, when fed CaMV[36].

An increasing number of scientists and doctors are also beginning to understand the connection between GMOs, glyphosate, and the rising number of cases of autoimmune diseases such as fibromyalgia, MS, rheumatoid arthritis, chronic fatigue syndrome, and others. According to the National Institutes of Health (NIH) more than 80 autoimmune diseases have been identified, with up to 23.5 million Americans being afflicted by at least one of them[37]. Evidence also suggests that GMOs and glyphosate are to blame for an increase in digestion-related autoimmune diseases, such as colitis, Crohn's disease, and irritable bowel syndrome, as well as other disorders like food allergies and intolerances[37-40]. This is due to changes in your gut bacteria levels, impairment of your mitochondrial communication system, as well as increased intestinal permeability, a condition more commonly referred to as leaky gut syndrome[40].

The consumption of GMOs *and* glyphosate has been shown to cause leaky gut syndrome by creating larger than normal openings in the epithelial lining of your intestinal tract and gut wall[39,40]. Like cheese cloth or a mesh screen, the epithelial lining of your digestive tract has tiny holes in it. This "cloth" or "screen" is in place to keep food and other substances in your digestive tract until full processing and waste removal is complete. A healthy digestive system breaks food down, extracts nutrients your body needs, and sends the nutrients into your blood stream via the epithelial lining, where they can be utilized[36]. However, when you suffer from leaky gut, the enlarged openings allow *undigested* food particles, proteins, and bacteria to enter your blood. These substances can travel to parts of your body where they don't belong and they are identified as foreign substances[40]. As a defense against these "intruders" your lymphocytes are activated and your body attacks the foreign invader with killer T cells and antibodies that come from B cells. This process creates inflammation in your body, a symptom of many autoimmune disorders. In addition, there are times when these antibodies can't tell the difference between you and the invader or your body fails to turn them off after they've done their job. Thus, your body literally begins to attack itself, and this is what is known as an autoimmune disease or disorder[40,41].

In addition, and like antibiotics, GMOs and glyphosate are known to affect gut symbiosis, altering the balance of healthy and unhealthy bacteria in your gut and weakening your immune system. These two toxic substances reduce the amount of Bifidobacteria and Lactobacilli in your bacteria colonies[39]. These beneficial bacteria have been proven to reduce inflammation in the body and lessen symptoms of celiac disease, a very serious and painful digestive disorder. As you'll read in a coming chapter, you need all the anti-inflammatory protection you can get to prevent virtually every type of disease.

So what does all of this have to do with animal consumption?

Factory farm animals are raised almost entirely on genetically modified crops. In fact, 98% of the GMO soy crops and approximately 79% of GMO corn crops produced in the United States are used solely for the purpose of feeding livestock. This means that, even if you're diligent about buying packaged foods marked as non-GMO and purchasing only organic produce grown without the use of pesticides, you're still consuming GMOs if you eat animals.

Humans aren't the only ones being affected by GMOs. For example, a long-term study determined that when pigs are fed GMO corn and soy up until slaughter, they suffer from serious conditions of the uterus, stomach ulcers, inflammation of the stomach and small intestine, cancer, hemorrhaging bowels, as well as several other conditions[42]. In addition, hundreds of published studies show that glyphosate and Roundup are dangerous and damaging to numerous species[43].

But what about meats marketed as grass-fed, pasture-raised or free-range? As of now, and as long as money is allowed to influence politics, we're relying on a government agency and government-employed inspectors to protect consumers rather than the interests of the agricultural industry. As mentioned in regard to cases of abuse and as you'll read in an upcoming chapter, the USDA doesn't have the best track record of placing public interest or animal welfare ahead of industry profits. Another concern, even if you are *truly* consuming pasture-raised animals, is the use of glyphosate-laden Roundup and/or other toxic chemicals sprayed on the grass, hay, or grains that these animals eat. Remember, pasture-raised doesn't necessarily mean that they were naturally fed or are GMO-free. So-called free-range animals are also often exposed to contaminated fertilizers in the form of manure from factory farms[44]. In addition, most pasture-raised animals are still injected with antibiotics and growth hormones[45].

One way to avoid *some* of the toxins in pasture-raised animals is to purchase organic meats. However, organic meat still contains substances that most consumers are unaware of such as methionine, a synthetic additive used to increase the growth of organic poultry[44]. Another drug commonly used in organic chicken production is gentamicin, an antibiotic employed to prevent chickens from developing a deadly herpes virus. Although antibiotics are prohibited in the production of organic animal products, a loophole has been exploited to circumvent the rule, whereby the antibiotic is injected into newly laid eggs[46]. It's important to remember, too, that *all* animals raised for their meat are subject to the same inhumane practices, abusive treatment, painful procedures, and violent slaughter as those raised on factory farms[47-51], and they still carry viruses and bacteria that can be passed onto humans.

Another important consideration involved in the farming of pasture-raised animals is the culling of wildlife, sometimes of endangered species, to protect herds from predators such as wolves, coyotes, and cougars. Not only does this involve the unnecessary killing of even more animals, but it has been proven ineffective and typically results in the attack of an increased number of farm animals[52]. Although the killing of wolves was outlawed in recent years, there's nothing to stop farmers from continuing with the practice in secrecy, and there are no laws to protect other such predators. In addition, you and I foot the bill for loss of livestock now that wolves have regained their endangered species status and are federally protected[53]. Unlike other business owners, who assume a certain amount of personal risk in regard to running their company, farmers receive taxpayer money to cover their losses.

As you'll read in the next chapter, even if we were to remove all of the animal rights issues and chemicals from the equation, there's still numerous scientific reasons to avoid the consumption of animal products.

II

You Be Illin'

While it's easy to understand that the drugs, hormones, and toxins found in animal products are dangerous for humans to consume, they're not the only cause for the growing number of diseases in the world.

Although these substances play a part in the proliferation and likelihood of disease by reducing our natural immune defenses, increasing our toxic load, and rendering life-saving medications useless, there's another underlying source of disease.

Based on a growing body of scientific evidence, what seems to play a central role in the development of many of the most deadly diseases is animal protein itself, as potentially deadly diseases such as cancer, heart disease, and diabetes have been traced back to elements within animal-based protein.

It's important to note, as you delve into this chapter, in relation to any report or study referenced, the term "red meat" includes beef, pork, veal, lamb, mutton, horse, and goat. The term "processed meat" includes any meat that has been salted, cured, fermented, smoked, or processed in any way to preserve the meat or enhance its flavor. Therefore, the processed meat category would include lunch meats, pepperoni, sausage and bacon products, hot dogs, and the like. Poultry, of course, refers to chicken, turkey, duck, goose, or any other type of winged animal.

As cancer rates continue to rise and the disease receives the bulk of media attention, it's easy to forget that the number-one killer in America is still heart disease. In fact, within the 10-year period from 2003 to 2013, one out of every three deaths in the United States could be attributed to some form of cardiovascular disease. On average, according to the 2015 American Heart Association report, one American dies from cardiovascular disease every 40 seconds[1].

Is animal protein related to this life-threatening condition? The answer is yes. A 2015 study[2] concluded that people with the highest intake of red and processed meat, respectively, had a 41% and 24% increased risk of stroke. In addition, those who ate the most eggs had a 41% higher chance of suffering a hemorrhagic stroke- that is, a condition in which a blood vessel becomes weakened and ruptures, causing blood to accumulate and put pressure on your brain. Numerous additional studies have resulted in similar findings and associate various forms of animal protein, particularly red and processed meats, with not just cardiovascular disease, but all forms of disease[3-8].

Even though red meat is often vilified and appears to be the most dangerous of the animal food kingdom, it's not the only animal protein associated with disease. Chicken, dairy, and eggs have also been directly linked to the occurrence of heart attack and possibly prostate cancer. There are many reasons for this connection, and studies show that a recently discovered toxin, trimethylamine N-oxide (TMAO), contributes to diseases of the cardiovascular system[9,10] as well as kidney disease[11].

TMAO is produced by the liver when meat-eating humans consume animal products. This is due to the interaction between our gut bacteria and nutrients found in animals, namely carnitine and choline. Not only does TMAO promote the formation of plaque in your blood vessels, but it also reduces your body's ability to excrete plaque-forming cholesterol. Although some of these same nutrients can also be found in plant foods, research confirmed that vegans are protected against TMAO production even when consuming carnitine, the reason being that those who follow a plant-based diet have gut bacteria that do not react to these substances in the same way[10]. Thus, when the two are combined, TMAO is not formed.

Studies indicate that the bacterial composition of your gut flora has a significant impact on the production of TMAO and therefore, an increased risk of cardiovascular disease when animal protein is consumed, once again, providing a warning against the use of antibiotics, GMOs, and other substances that alter the human microbiome.

TMAO researchers later discovered that consumption of carnitine produces something that poses an even larger threat to humans, gamma butyrobetaine, also called y-butyrobetaine (yBB). This metabolite produces at a rate 1,000 times higher than TMAO, when carnitine interacts with bacteria in the gut. Like TMAO, yBB accelerates the formation of arterial plaque, but it is generated from an entirely different species of bacteria. In addition, yBB can also be converted into TMAO when exposed to dietary sources of carnitine[12].

So, is it possible simply to reduce your intake of animal foods and still be protected? Studies of the microbiome suggest that the answer is no. This is so because gut bacteria are highly influenced by every meal you eat, and changes occur rapidly[13]. Even one meal of animal protein alters your levels of healthy gut bacteria, making you a candidate for diseases related to

TMAO and yBB production. In addition, research showed that TMAO levels remained elevated up to 24 hours following carnitine exposure, indicating that even one animal-based meal per day increases your risk of developing atherosclerosis[10].

In general, animal products increase dietary cholesterol levels in our blood stream. This cholesterol damages the inner arterial walls and causes inflammation. But because our bodies are amazing entities designed to self-heal, they go to work to make repairs with plaque.

Arterial plaque is a sticky substance that acts as a sort of putty, filling in holes and plastering over damage in the endothelial lining of the artery, much like you do with nail holes in the walls of your home. Sounds great, doesn't it? I mean, you just sit back and wait while your body does all the heavy lifting. It's like having a tiny handy man inside your body, on retainer, and on call 24/7, right? Well, sort of. Problems begin to occur when repeated damage is done, causing this layer of plaque to thicken, blocking large portions of an artery. Danger also arises when a piece of plaque breaks off and begins circulating through your blood stream, where it can get lodged in another artery or even a small vein. In either of these situations you're at great risk of a cardiac event such as a heart attack (when blood can't reach your heart), stroke (when blood and oxygen can't reach your brain or a blood vessel bursts inside your brain), or gangrene (when blood is unable to reach your extremities). Sadly, most people are completely unaware that they have blocked arteries until it's too late. Cardiologists state that the first sign of heart disease is often a fatal heart attack or stroke. However, unexplained fatigue and dizziness, shortness of breath (especially when exerting yourself), and erectile dysfunction[14] are early warning signs as well. In addition, and in women especially, neck, jaw, throat, back, or abdominal pain can also be signs of an impending cardiovascular event, while men are more likely to experience a pressure or tightening of the chest[15].

Then there's diabetes, the seventh leading cause of death in the United States, and the disease that was responsible for 1.5 million deaths worldwide in 2012[16,17]. Type 2 diabetes, once known as adult onset diabetes, is a disease that now affects young adults, teenagers, and even children. Of particular concern is the fact that when you have diabetes, your risk of additional health conditions increases substantially due to nerve and blood vessel damage caused by diabetes. In addition to blindness and amputations, which go hand in hand with unmanaged cases of this disease, diabetic patients often suffer from diseases of the cardiovascular system and kidneys[18]. According to the Centers for Disease Control and Prevention (CDC), one out of four people in the U.S. do not even realize that they have diabetes, and one out of three Americans are pre-diabetic, yet nine out of ten surveyed are completely unaware[19].

While numerous factors contribute to both type 1 and type 2 diabetes, the cause of this disease has been directly linked to the consumption of animal products. For example, in a meta-analysis following the progress of nearly 200,000 participants, scientists found that the consumption of red and processed meat increases your risk of type 2 diabetes. The research revealed that one daily serving of red meat, approximately the size of a deck of cards, increases the risk of type 2 diabetes by 19%. They also discovered that processed meat is far more dangerous, with the equivalent of just one hot dog or two slices of bacon accounting for a 51% increased risk of developing the disease[20,21]. Considering that most adults consume far more meat in one meal, it's easy to understand why the prevalence of diabetes is expected to double by the year 2030[22]. Another study, conducted over a 14-year period, attributes the acidic nature of *all* animal foods, including dairy, as the key to developing type 2 diabetes[23].

In addition to the nitrates found in processed meat, the fat and iron (heme) in animal meat causes pancreatic cell damage[24]. These substances can prevent insulin from attaching to receptors used to push sugar into your cells and provide you with energy. This is what is known as insulin resistance. As a result, your blood sugar levels rise and your pancreas continues to pump out insulin because your body mistakenly thinks that you don't have enough. This, of course, can lead to diabetes.

Likewise, impairment of pancreatic cells is fundamental to the progression of diabetes as these cells are responsible for digesting food as well as regulating the release of insulin and glucagon hormones into your blood stream. Together, these two hormones control your blood sugar levels. Thus, damage to pancreatic cells impairs your body's ability to balance your hormones and blood sugar levels, resulting in major health consequences including weight gain, internal inflammation, and finally diabetes.

It's important to begin eating plant foods as early in life as possible to prevent disease, as shown in a 2015 study[25]. During a 20-year follow-up, scientists confirmed that study participants with a high intake of fruit and vegetables in youth greatly reduced their risk of developing heart disease as an adult. However, the great news is that it's never too late and a plant-based diet not only has the ability to halt the progression of heart disease and diabetes, but it also has been scientifically proven to reverse completely these diseases and the damaging effects of animal consumption.

Doctors believe that plant-based diets are effective in curing diseases not only because they are void of *harmful* substances, but because they contain *beneficial* substances, including phytonutrients, chlorophyll, magnesium, fiber, and other such materials, most of which can only be found in plants.

Magnesium is particularly important in the prevention and reversal of diabetes and metabolic syndrome, as studies show that increased magnesium intake improves insulin sensitivity[26-28]. In addition, plant foods typically fall on the low end of the glycemic index, making them the best possible choice to control blood sugar levels. These facts explain the findings of three cohort studies that revealed that vegans had a 75% reduced risk of hypertension and between 47 and 78% reduced risk of developing type 2 diabetes, as compared with omnivores[29].

Scientists and doctors have documented the following health improvements for study participants and patients consuming a vegan diet, who had been diagnosed with cardiovascular disease and/or diabetes [30-35]:

Healing and repair of endothelial cells (the protective lining of arterial walls)

Increased diversity of gut microbiota

Increased number of microbiota

Improvement or reversal of erectile dysfunction

Improved insulin sensitivity

Improved renal function

Reduced carbohydrate sensitivity

Regulation and balancing of hormone levels

Reduction of LDL (bad) cholesterol

Reduction of visceral fat (abdominal fat that accumulates
around organs)

Reduced blood pressure

Weight loss

The vegan "side effects" listed above led to a reduction, or complete elimination of medications for participants in studies or patients adhering to the recommended dietary changes.

But what about cancer? Is it really caused by animal products? If so, can it also be cured in the same way as heart disease and diabetes? The answer is yes and yes to the two last questions. Please understand that in saying so, I completely recognize that this idea is controversial and that I may piss some people off. I get it. I've had far too many family members and friends who have lived through the ravages of cancer or who, sadly, have lost the fight and succumbed to this horrendous disease. It's admittedly difficult to believe that by switching their diet they could have been spared. But if we look at the fact that people are getting cancer much earlier in life, it seems obvious that something has *caused* this change. When my parents were in their 30s and 40s, they didn't have any friends or family members in the same age group with cancer. Yet many of my contemporaries, and some acquaintances even younger than I am, have been diagnosed with one form of cancer or another. This change suggests that the cause is environmental (something to which we're being exposed or are consuming) rather than genetic, because science tells us that genes cannot be altered so substantially from one generation to the next.

In *The China Study*, Dr. T. Colin Campbell details the longest and most in-depth nutritional study ever conducted in the history of mankind[35]. What makes this body of work and its information so reliable is that researchers, scientists, biologists, and physicians from around the world all came to the same conclusion without even knowing that other studies were being performed. Their findings confirmed that the intake of animal products by humans is a direct cause of cancer, heart disease, diabetes, and many other potentially deadly disorders. Most important was the discovery that these diseases were completely reversible by merely switching to a plant-based diet comprised of whole foods. In addition to the practical and medical experiences of the various physicians outlined in the book, Dr. Campbell performed a comparative analysis showing that when rats ate a diet consisting of 20% animal protein (well within the range of what humans consume on a daily basis in industrialized countries, and often even lower) cancer cells began to grow and tumors developed. However, when Dr. Campbell reduced the animal protein to less than 5% of total caloric intake in the same rats, the cancer cells began to die and tumors receded. He states in the book and in the related documentary, *Forks over Knives*, that you can literally "turn on and turn off cancer" by increasing or decreasing animal protein. This mind-blowing finding should provide hope to everyone who has ever felt fear and anxiety when faced with the prospect of a cancer diagnosis.

In addition to *The China Study* and other research conducted by well-respected scientists and doctors, two recent reports shook the meat and dairy industries with grim findings of a correlation between consumption of animal protein and cancer[36,37]. The results of these studies were also very disturbing to most people because they were conducted by independent and professional organizations with no affiliation or loyalty to any particular group or industry.

The first of the two reports was released in October, 2015, by the International Agency for Research on Cancer (IARC).

After reviewing 800 international studies, the IARC announced that they would be classifying processed meat as a Group 1 carcinogen, meaning that it is definitely carcinogenic for humans. They went on to state that red meat would be classified as a Group 2A carcinogen. The 2A classification signifies that this substance is *probably* carcinogenic to humans.

The IARC established that each 50 gram portion of processed meat (just over one-tenth of a pound) compounded and increased the risk of colorectal cancer by an additional 18%. They also stated that "these findings further support current public health recommendations to limit intake of meat." The report concluded that, while red meat is linked to colorectal, pancreatic, and prostate cancer, processed meat is a *direct cause* of colorectal cancer and is associated with stomach cancer. Based on its research, the IARC assessed that 34,000 annual deaths worldwide can be attributed to diets that include a high consumption of processed meats.

The second report, by the National Cancer Research Institute (NCRI), was published in November, 2015, after researchers studied and followed up with 500,000 men and women in the United Kingdom. This large-scale study determined that those who consume red meat four or more times per week were 42% more likely to develop colorectal cancer than those who consumed red meat less than once per week. In addition, those who ate processed meat two or more times a week had an 18% increased risk of being diagnosed with colorectal cancer as compared with those who never consume processed meat.

Additional studies have shown that men with a high choline intake-those who consumed the most meat, dairy, and eggs– had a 70% greater risk of dying from prostate cancer[38].

The correlation between cancer and consumption of all animal products, including poultry and seafood, has been studied as well. Research shows that specific animal products trigger various types of cancer. Therefore, particular types of animal food are related to higher mortality rates among those diagnosed with prostate cancer, while others may be more strongly associated with an increased risk of esophageal and breast cancer[39-41]. The most deadly cancer of all, pancreatic cancer, has been directly and substantially linked to red and processed meat, but not other forms of animal protein. In a multiethnic cohort study of nearly 200,000 people, participants showed a 50% increased risk from red meat intake, and a 68% increased risk of developing pancreatic cancer from processed meat consumption[42]. Similarly, red meat intake is associated with endometrial and lung cancer, and is believed to be the result of excess levels of heme[43].

Arguably, one of the most important findings of our time may explain why red and processed meat, in particular, instigate cancer and other diseases. In addition to the contributing factors previously mentioned, scientists have identified a sugar molecule contained in red meat, fish, and dairy, N-glycolylneuraminic acid (Neu5Gc). The human body lacks the ability to process Neu5Gc due to a mutation in our genes. However, scientists have established that prior to this mutation, which they estimate to have occurred 2.5–3 million years ago, humans *were* able to synthesize this molecule[44,45]. This raises the question, did human beings evolve into a species that does not require and should not consume these foods?

Neu5Gc is part of a family of nine-carbon sugars known as sialic acids (Sias). According to scientists, because Sias are found on vertebrate cells, they are highly involved in pathogen binding, inflammation, immune response, and tumor metastasis. All Sias are not created equal, however. Unlike Neu5Gc, other forms of Sias are extremely important to an infants' brain, and human breast milk contains high levels of beneficial Sias necessary for human, neuronal development[46].

Neu5Gc is present in all red meat, fish, and dairy, but this sugar molecule is most *abundant* in beef, lamb, and pork. Scientists began investigating the NeuGc cancer link after considerable amounts were found in human tumors. The molecule was also discovered on the cell surface of epithelial and endothelial tissues. The presence of this substance reveals dietary exposure because humans are unable to produce Neu5Gc. On the contrary, the human body contains several antibodies to protect us from this sugar molecule.

Although other species can synthesize Neu5Gc with ease, it is regarded as a foreign substance in your body. Thus, when you consume these animal substances inflammation-promoting antibodies such as IgC, IgM, and IgA are released in an effort to protect you. Likewise, in studies involving mice, this "nonhuman acid" caused inflammation, and long-term exposure resulted in a five-fold increase in carcinomas. As chronic inflammation is the foundation for all disease, scientists believe that this sequence of events is what ultimately leads to disease within humans. This provides an understanding of why those who consume the most animal products have a higher incidence of disease, particularly cancer, atherosclerosis, and autoimmune diseases.

Given the human brain's affinity for Sias scientists question the long-term effects of Neu5Gc and speculate if this is the source of neurodegenerative disorders such as dementia, Alzheimer's, and multiple sclerosis[44-52]. A link between Neu5Gc and thyroid disease may also exist as studies reveal that those suffering from hypothyroid and Hashimoto disease have much higher levels of Neu5Gc antibodies in their system[53].

Research has been completed to assess the impact of Neu5Gc on Kawasaki disease, a devastating pediatric heart disease that causes inflammation of the coronary arteries and can lead to aneurysms and heart attack in children. Scientists found Neu5Gc in Kawasaki patients, leading one to believe that this dangerous molecule is being transferred in utero. In addition, research in the U.S. has shown that Neu5Gc increases when a child reaches one year of age. This is associated with a change in dietary habits, from breast milk to dairy-based infant formula and the introduction of other animal products such as cheese and meat[44-53].

In regard to processed meat and its relation to cancer, evidence points to N-nitroso compounds (NOCs). High concentrations of these DNA-damaging carcinogens are found in food such as bacon, pepperoni, sausage, and hot dogs and derive from the nitrites and nitrates used in the processing of the meat[52]. Consistent with human studies, animal-based research confirmed cancer in 39 different species resulting from NOC intake[54]. Although the primary contributor, processed meat products are not the only source of NOCs. Studies indicate that heme (iron), found in all animals, incites the formation of NOCs[55]. While NOCs may play a central role in cancer, other components of processed meat products are related to diabetes, cardiovascular disease, and additional illnesses. Of primary concern is the high sodium and saturated fat content found in these products[56].

Arachidonic acid is another substance that acts as a catalyst for a litany of inflammation-based diseases. This acid, which is a naturally occurring compound in the human body, can be harmful in excess amounts and cause chronic inflammation when supplemented via dietary sources. According to the

National Cancer Institute (NCI), 10 out of the top 13 sources of arachidonic acid are animal related. Unlike other carcinogenic substances, the most damaging sources are found in poultry[57,58].

In addition to animal food itself, the way in which these foods are prepared can increase your risk of cancer. Dangerous compounds form within animal protein during the cooking process. Substantial amounts of these substances can be found in meat that is cooked for a long period of time (e.g., well-done) or at a high temperature, as with barbecuing, grilling, baking, or frying. Heterocyclic amines (HCAs) and polycyclic aromatic hydrocarbons (PAHs) have been proven to be carcinogenic, with studies showing that these compounds increase the formation of tumors in mammary glands, lungs, the colon, stomach, and prostate. Cancers of the breast, prostate, pancreas, colon, rectum, esophagus, lungs, and stomach have all been linked to HCAs and PAHs[59,60].

Considering the fact that lunch meats and eggs are staple foods eaten daily in many households, particularly in the United States, and that most people consume more than one serving of each of these foods in a single meal (e.g., bacon and eggs, pepperoni pizza, a bacon cheeseburger, etc...), it's no wonder that disease rates have skyrocketed over the past few decades.

The findings of international organizations, as well as those of independent physicians and scientists reemphasize the importance of a relatively new scientific field known as epigenetics, which involves the study of human DNA and, more specifically, how it can be altered or affected by outside influences. Through epigenetics, scientists are finding that they can either "write" on the DNA of humans, or erase coding that was thought to be hard wired in a human's DNA strand. Furthermore, scientists are beginning to understand that changes made to the DNA via lifestyle factors, can be passed on to future generations.

In essence, scientists are attempting to understand what many alternative-doctors and holistic practitioners have been saying for years. Namely, that disease can be caused by, and can therefore be healed by, diet, exercise, and other factors. Although this field is still in its infancy, existing studies have shown great promise and indicate that, although a human being may have a genetic predisposition to a specific disease, diet and lifestyle can literally alter those genes and change gene expression, preventing the disease entirely.

In addition to incorporating exercise and avoiding known carcinogens, nutrients and dietary compounds such as organosulfur, folate, polyphenols, isoflavones, selenium, isothiocyanates, vitamin D, and lycopene, have been proven to have a powerful impact on the epigenome and, therefore, the prevention or reversal of diseases[61,62]. In regard to cancer, scientists have proven that the processes that normally occur during carcinogenesis are hindered when cells are exposed to these substances[63]. Concentrated amounts of these nutrients can be found in plant foods and are, with one exception, absent in animal-based foods. The exception to this rule is vitamin D, which is more abundant in animals. However, the human body has the ability to self-produce vitamin D via direct sunlight. Vitamin D can also be obtained from mushrooms that have been exposed to high intensity ultraviolet light, morel mushrooms, fortified non-dairy milk, and vegan supplements[64,65].

How exciting is it to know that we can control our health outcome and override or turn off our negative genes? The best news of all, however, is that we can also turn *on* our good genes. One example of this was shown in a five-year study of men with prostate cancer[66]. The results of this study proved that we can flip the switch on our healthy genes and actually increase our lifespan with a plant-based diet and exercise, which lengthens our telomeres.

Telomeres, best described as a cap on the end of each strand of our DNA, are responsible for protecting our chromosomes and genes from damage, and for keeping them from touching and fusing together. Above all else, the length of our telomeres determines how long we'll live and how *well* we'll live because short telomeres are associated with osteoporosis, stroke, cancer, cardiovascular disease, diabetes, certain types of dementia, and other ailments. The aforementioned 2013 study, conducted by Dr. Dean Ornish, established scientific evidence that diet and lifestyle trump bad genes and that you can literally reverse the aging process with a vegan diet and minimal exercise.

While gene expression is immensely important in determining the root cause of one's propensity for disease, and the potential for preventing those genes from kicking in, it's not the only piece of the puzzle with which we need to be concerned. The consumption of animal protein has additional consequences that contribute to or directly cause health issues. One such contributing factor is the way in which animal protein impacts the pH level within your body.

To remain alive, your body must maintain a neutral pH level of 7.35. Animal foods cause your blood stream to become acidic, disrupting your pH level, and causing a condition known as metabolic acidosis. Although many have pointed to this condition as a contributing factor in osteoporosis, several studies provide evidence showing that the two are unrelated and that excess levels of calcium found in urine do not actually come from the human bone. Rather, the high volume and increased level of calcium is a by-product of animal protein itself[67,68]. However, researchers *have* discovered a link between animal protein and loss of lean muscle mass[69].

As mentioned, your body is innately protective and far more intelligent than even the most advanced computer system. Therefore, it does whatever is necessary to keep you from dying. In the case of metabolic acidosis, scientists have found that your body neutralizes the pH in your blood by drawing amino acids from your muscle.

When you consume acid-forming foods such as animal products, the acidity level in your body rises. Thus, your muscles break down to release amino acids into your system and neutralize the acidic load. This, in combination with diminished hormone levels, is believed to be the cause of reduced muscle mass as we age. It is also considered to be a primary factor in muscle wasting, particularly in the elderly and those with kidney disease. As renal function declines, the elderly and renally impaired lose their ability to excrete a great deal of the acids resulting from an animal-based diet, indicating that it is even *more* important to follow a vegan diet as we grow older[69-71].

Studies have established that alkaline foods, such as those eaten on a plant-based diet, reduce metabolic acidosis and helps you maintain a neutral pH level. In addition, scientists concluded that alkaline foods improve muscle mass, increase growth hormone production, and improve the efficacy of certain types of chemotherapy drugs. In addition, foods that improve alkalinity boost the amount of magnesium within our cells, which is crucial for the absorption and utilization of vitamin D. These combined factors contribute to our ability to maintain strong bones and ward off osteoporosis[69-71].

Although metabolic acidosis may not directly cause osteoporosis, there are numerous ways in which animal products cause our bones to become porous. These same foods are also responsible for our vulnerability to disease, particularly cancer. One such way is by reducing the amount of vitamin D in our bodies, as well as by increasing estrogen levels. Increased serum calcium levels have been proven to suppress vitamin D production in our body. This is incredibly detrimental to bone density and the strength of our entire immune system[72]. A reduction in this vitamin is particularly dangerous in regard to disease because vitamin D protects us against many cancers. In fact, numerous studies have inextricably linked dairy consumption to cancers of the prostate, testicles, endometrium, bladder, and ovaries, and others show that countries with the highest dairy consumption have increased incidence of prostate cancer[72-79].

Not only does one have a higher likelihood of being diagnosed with cancer as a result of dairy consumption, but the chance of dying from the disease also rises. A 2012 prostate-cancer study revealed that whole milk products increased mortality rates by 49%[80]. Likewise, a 2013 study on breast cancer showed that dairy intake was associated with increased mortality rates in general, and that those consuming more than one serving of high-fat dairy products per day (e.g., cheese) were 49% more likely to die from breast cancer[81]. Similar findings were documented in a study comparing testicular and prostate cancer rates in 42 countries, in which the increased intake of cheese, animal fats, and milk was positively associated with elevated rates of cancer[82]. Similarly, another study confirmed an increased risk of up to 92% with high cheese intake. Of all foods tested, cheese, milk, baked goods, and lunch meats were most strongly correlated to the incidence of testicular cancer[83].

Childhood consumption of dairy is of great concern as studies concluded that those with the highest adolescent intake of dairy were more likely to be diagnosed with testicular and colorectal cancer as an adult[84-86].

Again, one of the contributing factors appears to be calcium. So how much calcium does milk contain? Cow's milk contains nearly four times the amount of calcium found in human breast milk[87]. Obviously, if the human body is made to nurture and fully grow our species to the best of its ability, our own breast milk probably contains the proper amount of calcium, and anything more than that is harmful. This is the perfect example of quality over quantity.

As mentioned, the consumption of dairy products is also associated with elevated estrogen levels in humans. An increased level of estrogen is considered a high risk factor for breast, ovarian, and prostate cancer, and according to Harvard Ph.D. and scientist Dr. Ganmaa Davaasambuu, dairy products account for 60–80% of all estrogens consumed by humans[88]. This is, once again, due to the inhumane methods and practices used in factory farming, where cows are milked approximately 300 days per year. Throughout most of these 300 days cows are kept pregnant and milked, even in the late stages of pregnancy. The problem is that in the later months of pregnancy cow's milk contains elevated levels of estrogen–33 times the amount found in a non-pregnant cow. This explains the connection between dairy and cancers of the reproductive system, which is highly influenced by hormone levels. Thus, it's imperative to maintain a healthy hormone balance to avoid this disease.

In addition to the potential for osteoporosis and cancer, studies have linked milk intake to the underlying cause of *all* disease, higher mortality rates, and premature aging. A 2014 study conducted by scientists in Sweden showed increases in the oxidative stress biomarker 8-iso-PGF2a and the inflammatory biomarker Interleukin 6 with increased milk consumption. When elevated levels of these biomarkers are found in human blood, they are key indicators of impending disease and premature aging. Based on all of the data, the Swedish study concluded that when milk consumption increases, so does the overall risk of death. The researchers also showed that high milk intake does not reduce the risk of fractures and osteoporosis, as the dairy industry would have you believe[89].

So what's the big deal about oxidation and inflammation? Oxidation is what causes cars to rust and cut apples to turn brown. So oxidative stress essentially means that you're rusting on the inside, a condition reflected on the outside in the form of wrinkles, sagging skin, and age spots. On the inside, it produces free radicals, which damage your cells and DNA, making you a likely candidate for cancer and other debilitating diseases[90]. Scientists also attribute neurodegenerative diseases such as Alzheimer's and Parkinson's to oxidative stress[91].

Inflammation in your body is *the* fundamental and primary cause of all major disease. It's important to note, too, that it doesn't take much milk to cause oxidation and inflammation, thanks to a sugar contained in dairy, called D-galactose. In fact, in research on mice, as little as 100 milligrams of D-galactose accelerated the aging process, incited inflammation and oxidative stress, and led to cognitive dysfunction, damage of hippocampal neurons, and neuronal cell death[92]. To put this into perspective, a dose of 100 milligrams given to mice is the equivalent of 6–10 grams consumed by a human, or just one to two glasses of milk. In research on humans, D-galactose, which is abundant in cheese, yogurt, and even lactose-free milk, has been directly linked to ovarian cancer. One such study showed that women who consumed the equivalent of four or more servings of dairy products per day had a 60% increased risk of ovarian cancer[93]. Although four servings of dairy may seem extreme, consider that the United States Department of Agriculture (USDA) considers the following to be one serving[94]:

1 cup of milk or yogurt

1½ ounces of natural cheese

2 ounces of processed cheese

Based on USDA serving sizes most people typically exceed one serving in a single meal, especially when consuming cheese. In addition, consumption of dairy products has increased over the years. According to the Center for Science in the Public Interest, annual cheese intake increased from eight to twenty-three pounds per person when comparing statistics from 1970 with 2010[95]. Over the same period of time, yogurt consumption grew as well. When you combine these figures with ice cream, shakes, milk, and dairy ingredients hidden in packaged and processed foods, it's easy to understand how one person could easily consume and surpass four servings of dairy per day. Is it any wonder that disease rates have escalated?

Dairy consumption has further been linked to chronic and potentially life-threatening disease due to its role in epigenetic changes and its ability to stimulate insulin secretion and increase serum levels of insulin-like growth factor-1 (IGF-1).

Obese individuals and those with diabetes are known to carry the Fat Mass and Obesity Associated gene (FTO). The FTO gene is highly affected by two substances found in milk, branched-chain amino acids (BCAAs) and glutamine. Studies provide evidence of BCAA and glutamine's ability to change the expression of the FTO gene, causing obesity, type 2 diabetes, neurodegenerative diseases, prostate cancer, and breast cancer. Research further revealed that dairy consumption increases prepregnancy body mass index (BMI) as well as gestational, placental, fetal, and birth weight. Furthermore, dairy intake during pregnancy may result in the child becoming an obese adult due to "permanent changes in appetite control, neuroendocrine function, and energy metabolism in the developing fetus." This is also the case with children fed dairy-based formulas as it can permanently alter metabolic, neuroendocrine, and immunologic programming[96-99].

IGF-1 is another component of animal protein that plays a significant role in the cancer equation due to its effect on hormone levels. Although IGF-1 is a naturally occurring hormone in our body, elevated levels are strongly related to the promotion of cancer growth and other diseases[100]. This is especially true in regard to cancers of the prostate, colon, rectum, and breast[101-105]. Not only can IGF-1 instigate cancer production but it stimulates the development of additional growth factors, such as vascular endothelial growth factor(VEGF). This is very dangerous because VEGF can cause the formation of new blood vessels thereby providing tumors with additional sources of blood, causing proliferation and metastasis[106].

Studies show that men with the highest levels of IGF-1 have a four times greater risk of being diagnosed with prostate cancer[107] and premenopausal women are up to seven times more likely to develop breast cancer[108]. Other studies show that those consuming the most animal protein and milk had higher circulating levels of IGF-1[109]. Dairy, in particular, has been proven to increase circulating levels in humans. This is due, in part, to the fact that dairy cows, especially in the U.S., are injected with Recombinant Bovine Growth Hormone (rBGH), a growth promoter that is banned in Canada and the European Union. This genetically modified growth hormone increases milk production and, at the same time, increases the level of IGF-1 in animals[110]. In addition to instigating cancer, rBGH, in combination with IGF-1, is believed to be the cause of increasingly earlier menstrual cycles and breast development in young girls, which places these girls at greater risk for obesity, insulin resistance, type 2 diabetes, and cancer later in life. The drug has also been proven harmful to animals, causing painful and debilitating conditions including lameness and infected udders[111]. Any way you slice it (cheese pun intended) it's not good. Both the growth hormones and IGF-1 are passed on to humans who consume dairy products and cows' meat, contributing to various health complications and potentially fatal diseases.

Another cancer contributor is casein, the protein found in milk and other dairy products. In a 2014 study, scientists found that 1 gram of casein increased the growth rate of prostate cancer cells by up to 228%[112]. Casein was also the protein used in Dr. T Colin Campbell's rat study, outlined in the book *The China Study*, showing a definitive correlation between consumption of this animal protein and cancer development[35].

In addition to deadly diseases, studies have connected the consumption of animal protein, and the resulting inflammation and oxidative stress, to chronic conditions long thought to be unrelated to diet, such as depression, bipolar disorder, and other mental health conditions.

An estimated 350 million people worldwide suffer from

depression, and all we have to do is turn on the television to understand that this problem is growing worse by the day[113]. The airwaves are continually filled with stories of mass shootings in the United States, and most of the perpetrators are reported to be suffering from some form of mental health condition that failed to respond to drug therapy. Such drugs, in fact, can even make the symptoms of depression worse[114]. Studies show that although *some* anti depressants may partially relieve symptoms, the underlying cause of depression, inflammation, is not treated by existing pharmaceuticals[115].

As far back as 1887, scientist Julius Wagner-Jauregg claimed that inflammation was one of the triggers of depression. His studies led him to the discovery that those diagnosed with depression had high levels of inflammatory markers in their blood stream. Recent studies confirm his findings and further prove the connection between inflammation and mental health disorders[115-122]. Not surprisingly, those with mental health conditions frequently suffer with additional health maladies tied to chronic inflammation, such as cardiovascular disease, cancer, diabetes, autoimmune diseases, obesity, asthma, allergies, and more[119].

For the most part, mainstream doctors have argued against the idea that diet is a contributing factor in mental health issues. However, their long-held position has been disproven by studies revealing that endotoxins are a major cause of inflammation. These findings establish a direct causal link between the consumption of animal protein and depression, because animal protein contains endotoxins.

Within a matter of hours after being injected with endotoxins, participants in a study showed a marked increase in IL-6 and TNF-a inflammatory markers[120]. Likewise, they began to experience depression and feelings of social disconnection. Interestingly, male participants were affected for longer periods of time, with feelings of social disconnection increasing over a six-hour period, whereas female participants were more likely to experience an intense sense of social disconnection within the first two hours after exposure. The endotoxin depression link was further confirmed through brain scans, which showed that the pleasure center in participants' brains did not react to pleasurable stimuli, a condition known as anhedonia. In addition, the disparity in anhedonia between participants who received the endotoxins and those who received a placebo was tremendous[121]. A study published in 2009 further supported the connection between endotoxin intake and depressive symptoms. The findings of the study revealed that exdotoxin administration produced a reduced desire for social interactions, suppressed appetite, increased fatigue, caused sleep disturbances and cognitive impairment[122].

The link between diet and inflammation has been well established, even in the absence of endotoxins. One study conducted in 2013 confirmed that diets containing soft drinks, refined grains, red meat, and margarine were "significantly correlated" with inflammation[123]. Additional studies show that anti-inflammatory diets increase lifespan by lengthening your telomeres. In a five-year follow-up, scientists discovered that a highly inflammatory diet significantly accelerated the loss of telomeres. Those consuming inflammatory foods experience telomere shortening at nearly twice the speed of those partaking in an anti-inflammatory diet[124].

To combat mental health disorders, scientists are studying the use of anti-inflammatory agents, which have been shown to reduce mental health symptoms, even in patients with schizophrenia[125]. However, doctors and alternative practitioners have successfully used plant-based diets to cure patients suffering from these conditions[126-128]. This is due to the anti-inflammatory effects of antioxidants, which can only be found in plant foods. In addition, unless a vegan diet contains a great deal of oil and processed food, it is void of inflammation-inducing substances typically found in standard, omnivorous diets.

Although many cases of depression can be cured with a plant-based diet, other diseases involving the brain are not reversible, and they are also linked to the consumption of animal products. One such disease is Variant Creutzfeldt–Jakob Disease (vCJD). This brain disease causes symptoms consistent with dementia, but it progresses at a much more rapid pace and is always fatal.

The majority of cases of vCJD have been diagnosed in the United Kingdom[129]. However, as of 2014 there were 220 worldwide cases of vCJD in more than a dozen different countries[130,133]. Doctors believe that patients are infected by cows carrying a prion protein that initiates Bovine Spongiform Encephalopathy (BSE), a condition known to cause Mad Cow Disease[131]. In addition to vCJD, prion proteins have been associated with fatal familial insomnia, Gertsmann–Straussler disease, Huntington disease, and Kuru, all of which have a 100% mortality rate, often within a very short period of time.

In 2012, the USDA confirmed that a California dairy cow was in fact infected with BSE. Although the infected cow was euthanized, the U.S. government allows the sale of milk from infected cows. The reason being that the USDA claims that humans cannot contract the disease from milk because BSE only infects a cows' brain and spinal cord. The Center for Food Safety reports that brain and spinal cord tissues are often found in highly popular processed foods such as hot dogs, bologna, ground and chopped meat, and products containing gelatin[132]. Consumption of these products may explain the 2014 vCJD-related death of a man in Texas, the fourth such reported case in the United States. However, the U.S. Government maintains that all vCJD cases and subsequent deaths were the result of meat consumption outside the United States[133,134].

So we've talked a lot about red meat, dairy, poultry, and processed meat products, but what about fish? Are fish a healthy alternative and safe source of protein?

Studies have resulted in conflicting data. While some studies show that fatty seafood such as salmon have been proven to reduce chronic inflammation and aid in weight loss, others link consumption of seafood to an increased risk of diabetes and heart disease due to the high levels of saturated fat found in some sea animals[135-138]. Additional studies have focused on mercury contamination in seafood and the role it plays in creating DNA-damaging oxidative stress[139]. The data on cancer are also mixed as some studies report protective benefits against colorectal cancer, yet others cite seafood as a contributing factor in breast cancer[140,141].

Adding to concern about seafood, a CNN report stated that the United States imports approximately 90%, with the majority coming from aquafarms in China[142]. The FDA, however, claims that seafood imports account for only 80% of U.S. consumption, but they do admit that China is the third largest exporter of seafood to the U.S. Regardless of the actual figures, what makes this alarming is the FDA's 2016 warning that antibiotics and chemicals have been found in seafood from China, including catfish, basa, shrimp, dace, and eel. These potential toxins have not been approved for use in food in the United States and may pose serious health threats[143].

There are also other important factors to consider in relation to seafood consumption. Given the Fukushima radiation disaster, the runoff of waste, glyphosate, and medications from factory farms, and all of the known oil spills, it's clear that the oceans are overrun with toxic contaminants, which end up in the fish you consume.

Another concern in regard to seafood involves what the fishing industry refers to as "bycatch". This is the unintentional killing of highly intelligent sea animals. Each year more than 650,000 dolphins, whales, sea lions, and other marine mammals are unintentionally ensnared in nets meant for fish. Sadly, they are either left to suffocate or they're crushed by winches on the boat. Although the United States implemented new rules in 2015 to end these atrocities, there's simply no way to know if seafood suppliers are being forthright[144]. As with abuse of land animals, you have to catch perpetrators in the act to take action. In addition, these rules only apply to U.S. seafood imports. Other countries would need to implement their own similar laws or rules.

Scientists also are warning that we have depleted our oceans. According to a 2015 report compiled by the World Wildlife Fund and Zoological Society of London, as of 2012 and compared with 1970, marine life declined by 49%. The report further states that "humanity is collectively mismanaging the ocean to the brink of collapse." The current pace of large-scale fishing operations means that certain forms of sea life will not regenerate quickly enough and that we are causing species extinction[145].

As an alternative, you may be tempted to begin consuming farm-raised fish. However, I must warn against this, as these animals are also fed GMO grains. Not only are GMOs extremely hazardous to our health, as you've now read, but grains in general are also a completely foreign substance to fish.

In addition, fish are often dosed with toxic substances to enhance their size and color and, as mentioned, they are subject to many contaminants in the ocean. According to the Environmental Working Group (EWG), a non-profit consumer protection organization, seven out of ten farmed salmon purchased in U.S. grocery stores tested positive for polychlorinated biphenyls (PCBs). The seafood was sourced to factory farm-type facilities in Canada, Iceland, and the United States[146].

PCBs, which were banned in the U.S. decades ago, are known carcinogens. In addition, in human and animal-based tests, PCBs have been shown to disrupt thyroid levels, cause immune system damage, low birth weight, nervous system damage, neurological development deficits, liver toxicity, and elevated blood pressure, triglycerides, and cholesterol levels[147]. Based on statistics gathered at the time of the 2003 investigation, EWG estimated that an adult who consumes farmed salmon more than once per month has an "excess lifetime cancer risk of more than one in 10,000." It's important to note, however, that farmed salmon are not the only source of PCBs. The Office of Environmental Health Hazard Assessment in California website states that, in general, fish and shellfish contain PCBs and that spills, leaks, and improper disposal methods are the primary sources of contamination[148].

Fish bred on farms also receive vaccinations and antibiotics, and are exposed to pesticides as a means of reducing infectious disease, fungi, and parasites[149]. Scientists claim success in using vaccinations to treat conditions such as the pancreatic necrosis virus, salmon anemia virus, lymphocytic disease virus, and the Novirhabdoviruses[150]. However, due to the somewhat new and fast-growing industry of seafood farming, scientists are struggling to keep up with emerging and evolving pathogens[151]. The vaccines that do exist are often *made* from bacteria and viruses and, as a result, internal organ damage, abdominal lesions, autoimmune reactions, reduced growth rates, and forms of peritonitis have been reported as side effects[152]. While some of these drugs and toxins have been reviewed and proven unsafe for humans, as with pesticides, the majority of these chemicals remain untested to determine the long-term consequences of human consumption. It has also yet to be established whether farm-raised fish offer enough benefit to human health to off-set the potential risks.

When you consider all of these facts, it makes far more sense to get your anti-inflammatory Omega 3s from flax, chia, walnuts, hemp, and other plant-based options. The easiest way is to throw a handful of nuts or seeds in with a smoothie or non-dairy shake. An added benefit of these Omega 3 options is protection against heart disease, gallstones, inflammation, type 2 diabetes, and cancer, particularly of the breast and prostate.

12

Planet Earth

Like humans, our earth is becoming ill.

Educator and founder of the world's largest nutrition school, Joshua Rosenthal once said that even if meat were the perfect food for humans, we would still need to limit our intake. This is because our planet is in jeopardy, in large part, due to the harmful effects of methane emissions, deforestation, and the over-consumption of water used to raise animals.

The WHO released the findings of a study they conducted stating that in 2010 nearly a fourth of the planet's greenhouse gas emissions (24% to be precise) were the combined result of crop cultivation, livestock, and deforestation[1]. As of 2011, the United States and China were responsible for 44% of global emissions. When you consider that these two countries are also two of the top producers of animal products, and that the majority of crops in the U.S. are GMO corn and soy grown to feed livestock, it becomes clear that all emission roads lead back to animal production.

The WHO statistic is especially striking when you compare it with the finding that only 14% of greenhouse gases can be attributed to the burning of fossil fuels for *all* of the transportation methods on the planet.

Even if we simply reduce the number of livestock being raised for food, it's highly unlikely that would fix the problem, because the methane released from cow manure is far more destructive to the environment than even carbon dioxide from vehicles. The reason being that methane is approximately 30 times stronger than carbon dioxide in regard to trapping heat[2]. The world's population is expected to grow by one billion people over the next 15 years, according to the United Nations 2015 population report[3]. Of course, with more people comes more consumption, and factory farms are already operating at a pace that is unsustainable, and with consequences that threaten the continuing existence of the human race.

The situation is dire and is causing widespread damage due to the fact that cows alone produce 130 times more waste per year than all humans. Moreover, unlike human waste, animal waste is untreated and often finds its way into our water sources, killing off marine life and creating what are known as aquatic "dead zones." According to a 2014 report, there are more than 400 such dead zones throughout the world, primarily caused by agricultural runoff in the U.S. and Europe[4].

Consider too that an estimated 300 million tons of waste accumulate yearly in just the United States, producing emissions other than methane such as ammonia, hydrogen sulfide, and various other pollutants[5].

Hydrogen sulfide is a potent airborne contaminant and a by-product of hog farms. Low-level exposure to this toxin produces flu-like symptoms and high exposure has been proven to cause brain damage[6]. However, government "protection" agencies repeatedly fail to do their job. This failure was the basis for a lawsuit filed by the Environmental Integrity Project (EIP) and the Humane Society of the United States (HSUS). The lawsuit contends that U.S. residents are at great risk due to extreme levels of ammonia and hydrogen sulfide produced by factory farms. One Iowa resident stated that her family is forced to leave their home for "days at a time" when the toxic emissions are "at their worst," leaving her husband unable to breathe. EIP and the HSUS petitioned the Environmental Protection Agency (EPA) in 2009 and again in 2011, requesting that they investigate and intervene in regard to factory farm air pollution. However, requests were met with inaction, prompting the 2015 legal filing[7]. The HSUS announced their involvement in a similar lawsuit in July of 2015, involving ammonia emissions from a North Carolina factory farm that houses more than 8,000 pigs and produces approximately 38,000 gallons of manure and urine *daily*! Although required to do so, the farm owner failed to report "hazardous amounts of ammonia" during the five-year period leading up to the lawsuit[8].

Serious illness and even death is a very real concern when it comes to exposure of concentrated levels of ammonia and other noxious fumes from factory farms. Not only have large numbers of animals died as a result of this exposure, but farm workers have paid the ultimate price as well. In a 37-day study performed on piglets, scientists found that consistent exposure to ammonia resulted in respiratory disease and extinction of healthy nasal flora. Lengthier studies show that disease risk increases with extended ammonia exposure, as pigs studied for a five-week period were found to have bacteria in their tonsils as well as their nasal cavities[9].

So how much manure and ammonia are we talking about? I know that it's difficult to visualize thousands of gallons of manure (and maybe you don't really want to) but thanks to aerial footage taken in 2014, we know what we're up against. Documentary film maker, Mark Devries was able to obtain visual confirmation of a manure lagoon that was the "surface area of several football fields" at Smithfield Foods, one of the largest pork producers in the United States.

Deforestation is another dangerous component in this equation due to the fact that it removes our only source of clean air, because trees act as a sort of gigantic hepa filter by taking in harmful carbon dioxide and releasing oxygen. The combination of increased factory farming and deforestation is a recipe for disaster, one that most of the world is just now waking up to and trying to moon walk their way out of, while others continue to deny the reality of climate change.

In the Amazon alone, 136 million acres of rainforest have been cleared, often by burning, for the sole purpose of raising animals for human consumption. Obviously, this makes for a deadly combination, and it's also one of the leading causes of species extinction in South America; highly intelligent and social animals, are being uprooted and slaughtered at unprecedented rates to make way for livestock production. According to a 2006 report from the Food and Agriculture Organization of the United Nations, approximately 30% of the earth's surface is now used to grow crops for animal consumption and for the housing of farm animals[10]. Bear in mind that meat production has grown since that time and reports show a global upward trend for the future[11].

In addition to poor air quality, we also have to contend with water contamination from farming operations. Phosphorus, heavy metals, hormones, antibiotics, and nitrogen have been found in water wells, all the result of run-off and faulty manure lagoons. A perfect example of this occurred in 2005 when a manure tank ruptured, spilling three million gallons of cow manure into the Black River. It is estimated that approximately 280,000 fish were killed as a result, and one can only imagine how much of that sewage made its way into the tap water[12]. Accidents such as this are so prevalent that the environmental damage caused by animal agriculture costs a reported 34.7 billion dollars each year, in the United States alone.

Animal agriculture has been cited as a source of major nitrate pollution and was responsible for an unusually high number of spontaneous abortions in the state of Indiana in 1996. Authorities found that water wells had been contaminated by nearby factory farms.

In addition to the previously noted cancer risks associated with nitrates, high levels have also been proven to increase the risk of a potentially fatal syndrome in infants known as methemoglobinemia[7]. It seems, too, that history has taught the government nothing. After testing the well water in the farming areas of northeastern Wisconsin in 2008 and 2009, scientists found nitrates, fecal bacteria, and endocrine disruptors[13]. Like nitrates, endocrine disruptors can lead to cancer.

Citizens and environmental groups continue to fight, but the government seems unwilling to step in. In 2015, citizens and environmental groups petitioned their local government and the U.S. EPA after residents discovered that a Wisconsin dairy farm was contaminating the water supply[14]. A 2014 survey revealed that 70% of tested wells were contaminated with bacteria and that 30% of those wells contained "contaminants specific to cattle." Upon further testing, bacteria and nitrate contamination was discovered in more than one-third of the wells. The contamination is the result of spreading millions of gallons of liquid manure at Kinnard dairy farm. Kinnard, which was already estimated to generate 35 million gallons of manure annually, was given a permit to expand their operation from 5,822 to 8,710 cows by the end of 2017. Yet another example of government protection of corporate profits at the expense of individual citizens.

Sadly, this type of water pollution is not a rare occurrence. A 2014 report regarding the Missouri River Basin stated that "drinking water, aquatic recreation, and aquatic life" had been "compromised by high nitrate, bacteria, and turbidity levels," and cited "poor agricultural practices" as the cause. Of the 93 streams tested in Missouri, only three were fit to support aquatic life and only one stream was deemed safe for aquatic recreation[15].

As mentioned in a previous chapter, meat-eating humans are subjected to hormones, antibiotics, and other drugs used in standard farming practices. However, as evidence shows, even those who choose to consume a plant-based diet are ingesting and breathing in portions of these harmful substances due to air and water contamination. In addition, these contaminants not only pose a threat to humans, but to all forms of life, including our beloved companion animals and essential non-animal species.

To make the trifecta of planet damage complete, we have to look at the amount of water that's being used to raise and produce animals[16]. Believe it or not, between 34 and 76 TRILLION gallons of water are used each year in the feeding and production of livestock! You might wonder how this squandering of a precious resource is allowed to continue when some human populations in the U.S. have been faced with mandatory reductions in water consumption and other nations watch their children die due to lack of fresh water.

You may also wonder, as I have, what good it does to turn off the water while you soap up in the shower and then learn that it takes between 442 to 8,000 gallons of water to produce only one pound of beef and 1,000 gallons of water to produce only one gallon of milk[15]. Why so much? Because animals, such as pigs and cows, are large and drink a whole lot of water. Add to that the amount of water it takes to grow the crops of corn and soy that they're fed. Then there's the amount used to hose down waste and clean up after slaughter. Yeah, it's a lot!

Several issues allow this disparity to exist. One is that most environmental groups refuse to talk about livestock production and its relation to global warming because activists have been sued, and some even murdered, for standing up against Big Agriculture. This is particularly true in countries outside the U.S.[16].

Take, for instance, Sister Dorothy Stang, an American nun who lived in Brazil and was an outspoken advocate for protecting the Amazon against deforestation. In 2005 she was gunned down in the street by a hitman hired by a livestock producer. By 2011, Stang was just one of more than 1,000 people murdered for speaking out and taking action against the mass destruction of the rainforest. Unlike Dorothy Stang, most of the victims never received justice due to an overtly corrupt system and the deep pockets of land owners[17].

In addition, agricultural companies make large financial contributions to environmental groups with the expectation that they will remain silent about the environmental effects of factory farming[16].

Obviously, for a variety of reasons, you can't expect the government to speak up about this issue. As you'll read in the next chapter, a lot of it has to do with greed and conflicts of interest. However, one of the primary reasons why many government officials don't want to address the subject of factory farming and its relation to global warming is that it's a highly controversial subject. After all, telling people what they don't want to hear about habits they don't want to break is a great way to lose elections and tank your political career.

13

A Modern Myth

Right now, you may be asking, "What about protein? Don't we need it to survive?"

Yes, we absolutely, positively do need protein. However, you can survive, and even thrive, without protein from animals. The ironic thing is that you *cannot* survive and thrive without plant foods, yet most people limit or completely skip fruit and vegetables and load up on carbs and animal protein instead.

You may be able to adhere to an animal-rich diet and survive for a period of time, but you will suffer from a multitude of illnesses without the life-giving nutrients and disease-fighting compounds that only plants provide.

What many people are unaware of is that every plant food contains protein, in varying amounts. If you compare plant foods to animal foods, you'll find that some plants contain even *more* protein than meat, calorie for calorie. For example, broccoli contains more protein than steak, per calorie, and spinach is nearly equal to that of chicken and fish. It's difficult to comprehend why this information has been kept from the public, but it's just one of the ways in which we've all been fooled into believing that we *need* to eat animals or their by-products to build muscle or to sustain ourselves.

All anyone has to do to understand that plant protein is not only sufficient for human health but can also help to build incredible muscles and strength is to look at vegan athletes and bodybuilders such as Rich Roll, Carl Lewis, Robert Cheeke, Scott Jurich, Frank Medrano, Jim Morris, and many others.

The fact that you and I need protein to be healthy has been exploited by the food industry. It has used spin and hype to make the masses believe that more is always better, ignoring the scientific evidence regarding excessive protein intake and its relation to kidney damage and disease[1]. This lie has resulted in some sort of dead animal occupying the majority of most plates. All the while, vegetables, whole grains, and fruit have been relegated to the role of the meek sidekick, or worse yet, that character that you know is gonna die before the end of the movie.

Talking heads for the food industry have also perpetuated the myth that, unless you're getting your protein from an animal source, you won't be consuming all of the necessary amino acids. Therefore, they claim, that a vegan diet is inadequate for human health and survival. This fallacy was debunked long ago, yet in mainstream media you'll never hear about it or the dangers of animal protein. The fact is that plant foods contain all eight of the essential amino acids required by adult humans in varying amounts[2]. However, it's unnecessary to consume *all* of the required amounts of amino acids at the same time, as they're stored in your body's tissue and work in concert with each other over a 24-hour period. Therefore, it's nearly impossible *not* to consume at least the minimum amount of all essential amino acids each day unless you're just not eating *adequate* amounts of food or mono dieting–that is, eating only one type of food. Even in the latter case, simply eating large quantities of one particular food would increase your levels of all eight of the essential amino acids. However, I do advise against mono diets for extended periods of time because consuming a variety of plant foods better provides you with all of the various antioxidants, phytochemicals, vitamins, and minerals that the human body requires.

So why are we kept in the dark about the benefits and superiority of plant foods? The reason for this deception comes down to one thing–greed.

In her popular book *Food Politics*, Marion Nestle describes her eye-opening experience working with, and sometimes inside, the food industry[3]. As a nutrition policy advisor to the U.S. Department of Health and Human Services, Nestle witnessed firsthand the way in which those in the food industry used their influence and money to obfuscate and manipulate the truth about their products.

Industry lobbyists have employed intimidating tactics to strong-arm government officials into using generic phrases to deceive and confuse consumers. Toward that end, specificity is strictly forbidden. For example, Nestle provides an account of her first day on the job in managing the editorial production of the first ever Surgeon General's Report on Nutrition and Health. She was told that "no matter what the research indicated, the report could not recommend 'eat less meat' as a way to reduce intake of saturated fat."[3]

For decades, government reports could not specifically state that we should, "eat less meat" as a means to health. Because of this lack of clear-cut advice, consumers have largely ignored government nutrition reports and chalked it up to more scientific jargon that has nothing to do with them and their eating habits. The food industry giants know this. They know that most people will tune it out as white noise because trying to relate overused catchphrases to actual meals and specific foods takes too much time and effort. The result is that most people will go about their business and continue to eat as they always have. They assume (that darn word again) that, if there were something specific they shouldn't be consuming, something detrimental to their health, government officials would surely say so. This is just the kind of confusion and blind faith that food producers have counted on for decades to maintain the status quo and retain you as a customer.

Food manufacturers are also not above bribery to boost profits. In 2005 the non-profit advocacy group named Physicians Committee for Responsible Medicine (PCRM) and headed by Dr. Neal Barnard won a fight against the dairy industry and the National Dairy Council (NDC) for false advertising. The NDC had run an ad campaign promoting the notion that you could lose weight faster by consuming three servings of dairy per day. They claimed that this miraculous weight-loss method had been scientifically proven by Michael Zemel, Ph.D., at the University of Tennessee. The ads ceased when it was revealed that Dr Zemel was the recipient of grants totaling $1.68 million paid to him by none other than the NDC[4].

Conflicts of interest are not limited to the food industry and "scientific experts." They're also common in government. A quick review of the "USDA's Mission Areas" is all it takes to understand why government agencies fail to regulate food producers[5]. On the one hand, this government department is charged with the responsibility to "keep America's farmers and ranchers in business" and to use its resources for "domestic and international marketing of U.S. agricultural products." On the other hand, it is expected to "improve health in the United States," make certain that "the Nation's commercial supply of meat, poultry, and egg products is safe," ensure "the health and care of animals and plants," and "prevent damage to natural resources and the environment." As you've read in previous chapters, the latter of the two groups of responsibilities has *clearly* taken a back seat for years. Unless "we the people" stand up and demand that these contradictory responsibilities be handled by two separate entities, we will be forced to look over our collective shoulders to confirm that the fox is not guarding the hen house (farm pun intended).

Another reason for this duplicity is what has been called a "revolving door" between government and industry. Quite often, those who work for the corporations that produce pharmaceuticals, GMOs, and food products, are offered positions in government regulatory offices and vice versa. Many of these people know that if they just "play nice" and keep their mouths shut, they've got a cushy job waiting for them when they're ready to make a change and increase their salary. Some even move back and forth between the entities after several years.

Below, I've included a list of people who currently work with or for, or previously worked with or for, GMO manufacturers. This includes Monsanto, the largest manufacturer of GMO seeds and the company that developed and sells Roundup herbicide. Column three shows the positions that these same people held, or currently hold, within government agencies.

NAME	GMO Industry Ties	Government Position
Roger Beachy	Director at Monsanto Danforth Center	Director of the USDA's National Institute of Food & Agriculture
David Beler	Monsanto VP of Government & Public Affairs	Al Gore's Chief Domestic Policy Advisor
Dennis DeConcini	Monsanto Legal Counsel	US Senator
Linda Fisher	Monsanto VP of Government & Public Affairs	EPA Deputy Administrator
Mickey Kantor	Monsanto Board Member	Secretary of Commerce
Margaret Miller	Monsanto Chemical Lab Supervisor	FDA Deputy Director of Office of Special Nutritionals
Toby Moffett	Monsanto Consultant	US Congressman

NAME	GMO Industry Ties	Government Position
B Sesikeran	Trust Member of GMO & Pharma Funded, Int'l Life Sciences Institute	Chairperson for India's GMO regulatory agencies, RCGM & GEAC
Islam Siddiqui	Monsanto Lobbyist	Agriculture negotiator and Trade Representative
Michael Taylor	Monsanto VP of Public Policy	FDA Deputy Commissioner
Carol Tucker-Foreman	Monsanto Lobbyist	White House Appointed Consumer Advocate
Lidia Watrud	Monsanto Manager of New Technologies	USDA and EPA

Direct and indirect financial ties between industry and government officials also create a conflict of interest in regard to regulating companies and products. This matter was the subject of a 1999 lawsuit filed by numerous individual and group plaintiffs, including PCRM. The plaintiffs were victorious after the court ruled against the USDA in October, 2000, stating that the USDA had "violated federal law by withholding documents and hiding financial conflicts of interest." The lawsuit alleged and subsequently proved that six out of the eleven members of the Dietary Advisory Committee (DAC) had either current or recent financial interests in the meat, dairy, or egg industries. The plaintiffs further proved that others who took part in DAC meetings had working relationships with dairy companies, such as the Deputy Undersecretary of Agriculture who had a business relationship with Dannon[6].

It appears, however, that the tide may be turning and that certain departments of the U.S. government may actually be interested in protecting the citizens who pay their salaries. Either that or they're putting on a good show.

As of January, 2016, the USDA included wording in the updated and official U.S. Dietary Guidelines recommending that "individuals should eat as little dietary cholesterol as possible." Most shocking was the further statement that "dietary cholesterol is found only in animal foods such as egg yolk, dairy products, shellfish, meats, and poultry." OUCH! That one's gonna hurt.

Maybe this change was brought about by pressure from the American people after they read the IARC and NCRI reports on cancer and completed those easy-to-sign online petitions. Or perhaps, once again, it was the result of the incredible work of Dr. Neal Barnard and PCRM in filing a lawsuit over conflict of interest claims[7]. The lawsuit alleged that several Dietary

Guidelines Advisory Committee(DGAC) members had either financial or business ties to the egg industry with some receiving substantial research grants, as proven by documents obtained under the Freedom of Information Act (FOIA). The suit further cited that the DGAC used "egg-industry-funded research" to determine cholesterol guidelines and excluded additional scientific research showing the dangers of cholesterol. Apparently, the USDA and senate were conspiring to omit phrases pertaining to cholesterol levels when PCRM filed its lawsuit. Eyeaaaah, I'm leaning toward the lawsuit as the reason for this sudden urge to protect the people. Whatever the case may be, we should all be grateful that this life-saving information will finally be a part of the official record and consumers will no longer be left to decode the hidden messages.

Consumer advocates are cautiously optimistic about the new USDA guidelines and hopeful that this will have a positive effect on the foods that children consume, because the U.S. Dietary Guidelines have long dictated what is served in schools under the school lunch and breakfast programs.

Again, you will not see, hear or read a whole lot about this development in mainstream media because, as the saying goes, they have a dog in the fight. With rare exceptions the media outlets keep quiet about everything I've outlined in this book. To understand why, all you have to do is ask yourself two questions: (1) What industry/product is most advertised on TV and in magazines nowadays? and (2) Who has the most to gain by keeping you and me sick? Obviously the answer to both questions is the pharmaceutical industry.

As you know, television stations and magazine companies make money by selling ad space in the form of commercials and print ads. Media professionals know that, if they were to allow coverage of the *real* reasons why so many people are sick and in need of medical treatment, or of how animals are treated on factory farms and the environmental damage caused by feedlots, many people would be outraged and stop consuming animal products. That would spell disaster for many of the most profitable industries in the world–healthcare, pharmaceuticals, food, and media.

Obviously, greed and deception are very real concerns when it comes to political oversight, but I do believe that there are still a few decent politicians that actually care about us–their constituents. The problem is that they are a minority. Another consideration we need to keep in mind is the fact that government officials are simply human beings prone to mistakes and misstep. As you've now read, in regard to BLV, antibiotic resistance, and many other health threats, the government doesn't know what they don't know. Even if they want to, they cannot protect us against threats that they're unaware of. If they couldn't anticipate that the overuse of antibiotics in livestock would lead to worldwide immunity, then we have to assume that they lack the knowledge and experience necessary to predict the consequences of their lax policies and others' greedy actions. Therefore, we need to be vigilant and take action to protect ourselves and those we love. The good news is that it seems that more and more people are doing so, with grassroots movements to return to natural foods and common sense.

So we're catching on in advanced nations, and the U.S. government appears to be stepping up to provide truthful and explicit guidelines for once. But what about the people in developing countries, especially those who rely on imports from the United States? One such country is Haiti, and as I learned from my Haitian friends, their families are now consuming more animal products from the U.S. than they are from their own country. This change is disturbing when you consider all the chemicals, drugs, and genetically modified ingredients in these products. Apparently, however, as in many countries, the people of Haiti regard the purchase of American products as a sign of wealth and status. They're impressed by the exceptionally large chicken legs and breasts, which are reported to be two to three times the size of chicken parts from Haitian farms.

The exporting of our culture and food is nothing new, though, as most industrialized countries at some point begin to emulate the eating habits of Americans and import our products and fast-food franchises. While imitation is considered to be the sincerest form of flattery, it appears that it's also very dangerous. Everywhere our Standard American Diet (SAD) and agricultural products go, our diseases follow. This has been the result in every country where the dietary pattern shifted to a more "Western" way of eating. Time and again it has been shown that those who adopt a typical American diet begin to gain weight, develop diseases, and experience fatigue, just like a majority of the population in the United States[8-11]. It seems, then, that we're exporting myths and disease as much as food.

This concept was most clearly shown in *The Blue Zones* by Dan Buettner[12]. In his book, Buettner detailed the findings of his team's extensive research regarding specific regions of the world and populations with an exceptionally high number of healthy centenarians. What they discovered, among other things, is that these individuals consumed the traditional and largely plant-based diets of their ancestors. This allowed them to live up to and beyond 100 years of age, free from disease and the mental and physical deterioration so typically seen throughout the rest of the world. Often these centenarians were healthier than the younger generations in their geographical area. This was due, in large part, to the fact that these young people had abandoned the diet of their ancestors and adopted a more "Western" diet, consuming animal products at each meal and taking part in the growing popularity of convenience and fast foods.

Because the world follows our lead so often, it's even more important that the people of the United States move toward a healthier and more sustainable plant-based lifestyle.

14

Family Affair

While it's clear that there are many mechanisms through which animal protein causes disease, you may still be hesitant about shifting to a vegan diet.

The thought of making this change may seem monumental and overwhelming. I totally get it! Hell, I grew up working in my parents' Italian deli and brought sandwiches with me to school almost every day. It doesn't get more animal-based than that. So I can completely relate to what you may be thinking and feeling. I remember when the thought of not eating meat at every meal seemed strange and abnormal to me. It just didn't seem possible, especially considering doing it for the rest of my life. However, now it's second nature.

I understand that just the idea of removing this "staple" from your diet can be daunting if you don't know where to start and what to do. After all, it's chicken with this and steak with that in most households. That's exactly how it was in our household, but I can attest that it's easier than you think and you'll be glad you made the change. In fact, many people (myself included) wish they had done it sooner, after they realize how much better they feel.

The first thing I suggest is that you try to appreciate and embrace the need to protect yourself and your family. No one else is going to do it, and when I truly understood this fact I began thinking of food choices as one more responsibility I had to keep my children safe and teach them the basics about life and potential dangers in the world. I now view it as no different than teaching them to look both ways before they cross the street or not get into a car with a stranger.

The dangers of consuming animal protein became very concrete for me when I realized that placing a piece of animal flesh on my child's plate was like a slow poisoning. One serving may not be lethal, but over the course of time consuming that animal protein is tantamount to ingesting a drop of drain cleaner with each meal.

Remember too, it's not just about removing the dangerous foods, but also about leaving more room on your plate and in your stomach for foods that provide what your body requires to maintain homeostasis and increase the amount of enjoyable and productive time you have here on earth. It's about giving you and your loved ones the best chance possible for as many years as possible.

For decades study after study has scientifically proven that animal foods incite and perpetuate disease while plant foods, including spices, have the ability to prevent and/or cure disease, and to alleviate symptoms of a vast number of chronic conditions including the following[1-149]:

Alzheimer's

Arthritis

Autoimmune disease

Bipolar disorder

Cancer

Cardiovascular disease

Chronic Fatigue

Colitis

Dementia

Depression

Diabetes

Diverticulitis

Erectile Dysfunction

Fibromyalgia

Glaucoma

Insulin resistance

Irritable bowel syndrome/Inflammatory bowel disease

Macular degeneration

Metabolic syndrome

Multiple sclerosis

Obesity

Thyroid disease

In my brain I picture the Fruit and Vegetable Band in a singing competition and they're the final contestants up against the Meat Band. Broccoli is on the mic, and at the top of his lungs he belts out, "anything you can do, I can do better." Simon Cowell gives a standing ovation and announces that the Vegetable Band has "got the X Factor." Why? Because I have an over active imagination and because there's nothing in animal food that plant food and nature can't match or exceed. Conversely, animal foods are completely void of specific compounds and nutrients that are *essential* for survival and virtually every bodily function. Things such as antioxidants, chlorophyll, fiber, and phytonutrients are the only things standing between you and disease, yet they do not exist in animal meat. So, to eat animals is strictly a choice, not a necessity. Once you understand that, it will seem crazy to cause suffering and pain that serves no purpose.

As mentioned, I didn't come to realize this all on my own. In the beginning I watched documentaries about the food industry, about people who became vegans, about factory farms and the environment, and to my surprise my daughter began watching with me. She began sitting next to me on the couch, and before I knew it we'd be cuddled up together and crying or yelling (sometimes both) at the TV screen.

I suggest that you invite your family to watch such documentaries with you. Even if you have to promise them a favor in return, it's well worth it. Having the information come from a third party is the best way for you to share these messages with other members of your family. While it may be easy for them to tune you out and assume (there's that word again) that you're being dramatic or fanatical, seeing the images and hearing from experts open them up to understanding your commitment to change. And if they like to read, then by all means hand them this book.

Getting your family involved in the mission is also a great way to motivate your children (and hopefully your spouse - wink, wink) to help out in the kitchen. Meals will be prepared faster with their assistance, and if they're too young and not ready for knives (hopefully *not* your spouse), you can at least have them stir while something simmers, freeing you up for other tasks or a rest. You'll also be teaching them a basic but highly important life skill–how to cook. And you know what they say: "Give a man broccoli, and he eats for a day. Teach a man how to cook broccoli, and he gets to eat it for the rest of his life *and* keep his colon." Okay, maybe "they" don't say that, but *I* do.

There are a few documentaries and videos that I highly recommend. Some focus on the health benefits of a plant-based diet, others discuss the effects of our industrialized system of agriculture and how it's damaging our planet. There are also some that include information about the treatment of animals on factory farms, and its implications.

It's best to determine what each family member's "hot button" is and choose a movie that touches on whatever subject that may be. Children are more likely to care about the animals, while adults (especially men) are typically more compelled by health ramifications or consequences to the planet. However, everyone is different and you know them best, so use your best judgment.

I would also suggest that you view the documentaries ahead of time to gauge what is appropriate for your children based on their age and maturity level. After all, we want to effect change but not at the risk of scarring them for life and causing nightmares.

Many of these films and lectures can be found on YouTube and viewed for free. Others may be available on Netflix, Amazon Prime, or other streaming video services at minimal or no charge. Here's a list of my top choices:

Beyond Carnism (TEDx)

Cowspiracy

Crazy, Sexy Cancer

Dying To Have Known

Earthlings

Food Inc

Forks Over Knives

Live and Let Live

Peaceable Kingdom

Plant Pure Nation

Speciesism: The Movie

The Gerson Miracle

The Ghosts In Our Machine

The Witness

Vegucated

A question I hear frequently is, "How do you find the time to prepare a home-cooked vegan meal each night?" Yeah, I understand that too. In a world of dual-income families and kids with more social and academic obligations than ever before, it can be challenging.

One of the easiest things you can do is to cook double recipes on your day off and freeze half for a work night. You can also plan all of your work night meals in advance, do the shopping and prep some of your vegetables on your day off. Washing and cutting vegetables in advance will save you time on those busy nights. Just be sure not to cut them up too far in advance (more than two to three days ahead, especially for vegetables with a high water content), and always store them in the fridge in airtight glass containers. Buying mason jars by the case is perfect for this use.

And while I don't encourage a diet filled with packaged, processed, or fast food, I live in the real world and understand the necessity to incorporate some of these foods into your meals.

When life becomes chaotic and you're forced to grab a quick meal on the go there are several options you have. A smoothie or juice may tide you over, but if you're interested in a full meal, choose a restaurant or fast food chain that offers burritos, tacos, fajitas, salads, bowls, or wraps. These menu items can easily be made vegan by simply asking them to remove the meat and/

or cheese and to substitute those items with additional veggies, rice, and/or beans. Substituting avocado for cheese is perfect. It's an abundant source of protein and essential fat, and it can really satiate your craving for cheese. Asian cuisine also typically offers standard plant-based menu items such as cucumber rolls, California rolls made with faux crab meat, vegetable lo-mein or chow mein, and other vegetable-rich dishes. Be sure to ask, though, what kind of broth they use as a base. Often vegetable dishes are made with chicken broth. However, most restaurants are more than happy to substitute vegetable broth in your meal.

Whenever possible, prepare your meals at home to avoid GMOs, additives, and excess salt, sugar, and fats. Meat alternatives, especially, can serve as perfect transition foods while you're making the switch to a plant-based diet. Of course, you can continue to use these substitutes as you move forward in your vegan lifestyle, but it's best to increase your intake of whole-foods as much as possible. Real food, as nature created, will always give you the most valuable nutrients and in their most complete form.

Some popular meat substitutes are made by companies such as Boca, Beyond Meat, Gardein, Tofurky, and Starlite Cuisine. You'll find everything from breaded "chicken" patties and taquitos to ground "beef" and BBQ pulled "pork." One of my favorite brands is Beyond Meat. They make "chicken" strips, which are as close to the real thing as possible and work great in any recipe that calls for chicken or in a quick wrap along with lots of veggies and a healthy dressing. Beyond Meat also makes ground "beef" which is perfect for tacos, chili, meat sauce, or anything else you'd normally put ground meat in. The best part is that it's made with pea protein, so if you have an intolerance to soy or are trying to limit your intake, this product is ideal.

As for cheese products you can find some tasty "cheese," cream cheese, and sour cream alternatives made by Follow Your Heart, Tofutti, Miyoko's Creamery, Go Veggie, and other manufacturers.

I suggest reading labels closely and trying to limit your intake of soy protein isolates and soy oils as much as possible. Unlike the whole-food and minimally processed forms of soy such as tempeh, edemame, tofu, and miso, which have been shown to reduce cancer risks[111-127], soy isolates can have some detrimental health consequences. Instead, when possible, try to use convenience foods containing other forms of plant protein such as seeds, nuts, beans, hemp, and peas.

When it comes to making the transition, there are a few things you can do to get started without any research or hiring a coach. One thing that's simple yet effective is to try making your favorite meal without the meat. For example, one of my husband's favorite pre-vegan dinners was steak with a baked potato and grilled asparagus. I still make this dinner minus the meat. Instead, I make extra asparagus or potatoes, and if I don't have enough of those items I add a salad to the meal. This is an easy way to still get some of the tastes and textures you're used to while becoming accustomed to meatless meals.

Another thing you can do is to search through your old family recipes and ask your elders for any that they might have. You'd be surprised to discover how many older recipes are "accidentally vegan." This is due to the fact that many of our elders, especially those who have passed away, grew up during war-time and even during the Great Depression. They learned how to create meals without meat because it was too expensive to have on a daily or even weekly basis. In addition, factory farms did not exist then and meat products weren't transported all over the globe, as they are now. Therefore, meat products weren't widely available and meat consumption was minimal.

You may also discover that some of your dated family recipes contain animal protein in the form of butter, milk, or eggs. These are easy ingredients for which to find vegan substitutes, and you typically won't notice a difference in taste or texture.

The best vegan butter on the market is, hands down, the Earth Balance brand. They make tubs of a spreadable version, and they also sell "butter" sticks that are perfect for baking. Their products also offer variations in ingredients, including a soy-free option. I recommend this version, especially if you have a food intolerance to soy or have had issues with estrogen dominance, since soy can increase estrogen levels. You'll love these products regardless of which option you choose, and even the biggest butter or margarine lover won't be able to discern the difference between the real thing and Earth Balance's product.

There has never been an easier time in history to find great non-animal substitutes for milk. In fact, if you scan the milk section of any well-known grocery store, you're likely to find a half dozen options. Non-dairy milk has become extremely popular, and the type you use really is more about your personal taste than anything else. I tend to lean toward nut and seed milks, with my favorites being soy, cashew, and flax milk. In addition to these three, however, you can find rice, coconut, hemp, and almond milk just about everywhere. However, they each have distinct tastes and consistencies, with some being thicker than others. So if you're using one in a recipe, it's wise to taste it first to ensure that you like the flavor and that it's not too thick or thin. The mildest of the bunch are flax, rice, and soy, while the others have a tendency to dominate the flavors of a recipe.

Egg replacement can get a bit tricky. The thing about eggs is that they're used for various reasons depending on the recipe.

They can be used to help thicken or to add flavor or simply to bind ingredients together. In addition, some recipes call only for the yolk, while others require only the white of the egg. The easiest substitute is an egg-replacement product. There's a lot of competition in this market now, with brands such as Bob's Red Mill, Orgran, The Vegg, and others competing for your dollars. However, there's one absolute stand-out that's the closest thing to a real egg that you can get in terms of texture, look, and taste. It's made by the Follow Your Heart brand, and it's called VeganEgg. The best part about this product is that, unlike other replacement products, it is meant to be a faux egg and can be eaten on its own *or* used in recipes. This product makes such authentic "eggs" that you can scramble them and make an omelet. In addition, they're made from algae flour and algae protein, so you're getting a plant-based product that's packed with life-giving micronutrients.

As a side note, keep an eye out for additional algae-based products in the near future because food companies are currently developing healthier milk and oil products by using this nutrient-dense ingredient.

Here are some guidelines to follow if you'd prefer to make your own egg replacement or want a whole-food option rather than a packaged product that may contain preservatives or other ingredients.

Egg Substitute	Substitution For One Egg
Ground flax seeds work best as an egg alternative in baked foods This is a perfect replacement in muffins, cookies, and sweet breads (ie: banana bread, corn bread, etc) Golden flax seeds are better than brown flax seeds that may be visible in the final product	Grind flax seeds just prior to use Mix one tablespoon of ground flax seeds with three table-spoons of water Whisk together and let stand for five minutes. Then use as you would an egg
Bananas provide a great deal of added moisture to recipes, along with a strong flavor, so use with caution You might need to reduce the other liquids in your recipe with this option	Completely mash 1/4 cup of ripe banana and use as you would an egg
Tofu works in dense foods, such as brownies or pound cakes, but is too thick and heavy for light, fluffy foods	Puree 1/4 cup of tofu and use as you would an egg

It's important to note that, when using ground flax seeds, you will need to store any unused portion in an airtight container in the refrigerator and only for two to three days. Although whole flax seeds remain edible for long periods of time, ground flax seeds become rancid quickly, even in the fridge.

"Great," you say, "but where can I find recipes to use these ingredients, Gina?"

I'm so glad that you asked!

To find just about every plant-based recipe under the sun and ways to use these great animal-product replacements, please visit my websites, 360HealthConnection.com or Proud2BV. com.

In addition to my own vegan recipes, you'll find resource pages complete with hundreds of links to vegan websites, recommended reading, and plant-based resources and products. The lists I've compiled are extensive, so take your time and try not to get overwhelmed.

15

Hero

The third turning point in my 180, occurred when I learned of, and virtually attended, the Food Revolution Summit. This ultimately led me to the point that I'm at now with a new career and burning mission, as though someone came by and pushed my "on" button for the first time in life.

Throughout my journey I've been blessed to find incredible mentors. Some have been found in the pages of best-selling books and through my professional studies. However, some of the best resources are the ones that I've stumbled upon by accident. These are the ones that I'd find a mention of embedded in a blog post or news article. The Food Revolution Network was one of those incredible finds.

This organization, founded by genuine visionaries John and Ocean Robbins, opened my eyes and mind to things that I couldn't believe I had never known. This is where I first learned about the dangers of GMOs and about how our food system has been taken over by companies that fill our bodies with toxins and addict us to their commercial products, and SO much more! Through the Robbins' free, online summit I learned of additional resources that enabled me to continue along my path. For this reason stumbling upon the Food Revolution Network was the single most important discovery of my professional life and for my healing success. The speakers included a plethora of activists and medical professionals, as well as industry, health, and food experts, who freely shared their knowledge, insights, and research. Because of their infectious desire to share the truth and their sincere wish to help others, I knew that I had to become part of this movement.

So began my mission, and I availed myself of every morsel of information the speakers provided. I became familiar and affiliated with websites, activist groups, and protection organizations. I scoured the pages of books and watched every recommended and linked video. I had found a way to stay the course and not feel deprived while my health soared.

As mentioned at the end of the preceding chapter, you can find links to anything and everything plant-based via my websites. However, I'd like to share here a few of my favorite sites, including some that are health-related but not necessarily vegan-specific.

These are the websites of people and organizations that have had a tremendous impact on my life and health.

Carnism.org

CenterForFoodSafety.org

DoctorKlaper.com

DrEsselstyn.com

Engine2Diet.com

EWG.org

FoodRevolution.org

ForksOverKnives.com

KrisCarr.com

OrganicConsumers.org

OrnishSpectrum.com

PCRM.org

ResponsibleTechnology.org

RobynObrien.com

TheTruthAboutCancer.com

16

Feelin' Good

With help from people for whom I have tremendous respect and admiration, I was able to heal my body and I felt, and continue to feel, absolutely amaaaaazing!

Just a few short months after abandoning my omnivorous diet, my health was completely transformed. It was as if I had gone in for a body overhaul and was given a new engine.

Lab work and a follow-up visit to the hormone specialist revealed that my once perimenopausal body had returned to its premenopausal state. The doctor asked me what I had changed as she reviewed my blood work and explained that my hormones had returned to healthy levels, all without the use of hormone replacement therapy. When I told her that I had cut out all animal protein, she replied, "Keep doing whatever you're doing because you've reversed the aging process." Is that incredible or what?

Not only were my hormones back on track, but I was sleeping peacefully throughout the night, and my allergies, asthma, and cystic acne had all but vanished. No longer did I need to wash every single piece of my bedding weekly, for fear that dust mites would send me into a two-week sinus infection. I could also actually wear v-neck and open-backed clothing again without being embarrassed by my acne-riddled chest and back. I had energy to spare and no longer needed a cup 'o joe in the afternoon. The seasonal depression that had plagued my holidays forever was a thing of the past, and I realized that I hadn't been sick since the horrendous lung infection that I suffered with seven months earlier.

This was insane! I had never gone six whole months without an illness in my adult life! Although I never dreamed it was possible at that time, I would go on to enjoy more than three consecutive years without a single illness—not a cold, not a flu, nothin', zip, nadda. And this was while everyone around me was getting flu shots and then *still* coming down with fever, chills, aches, and pains.

Feeling better than I did twenty years ago, what I've come to understand is that life can be incredible and rich and abundant in all ways.

I discovered the secret cause of disease, and I came to recognize that we can choose not only how we want to live but also, for the most part, how we wish to die. We can either die peacefully in our sleep at a ripe old age, maybe even as a centenarian, or we can die slowly each day in pain and exhausted by chronic illness and disease.

I was reminded, and will never again forget, that all living beings experience pain, joy, pleasure, and fear and that they all love their offspring and want to live as much as you and I do.

Most importantly, I found evidence of the purpose of life–namely, to use our unique talents, challenges, experiences, and abilities for the greater good of all.

Toward that end I've rededicated my life to helping people get healthy, while saving animals and the planet along the way, and I couldn't be more excited about the difference I'm making in the world. I now can honestly say that the work I am doing feeds my soul, and that's far more rewarding than any amount of money in a bank account.

17

Come With Me Now

I used to wonder why God or the universe or whoever runs this place would make me allergic to animals and then put such a HUGE love for animals in my heart. It seemed like a cruel joke.

While at a party at my best friend's house, I remarked on this cruel and unusual punishment and finally got an answer that made sense. I was told that the Haitian people believe that it is the devil, not God, who places such challenges within us. He does this to inflict pain and to instigate conflict in our hearts and minds. They believe that he does this to see whether he can cause us to act against our instincts to do the right thing or shut down our capacity for love, acceptance, and compassion.

So perhaps, this is a test of all mankind.

WHAT THE FORK?

"You may choose to look the other way,
but you can never say again
that you did not know."

~William Wilberforce

Will we act against our base nature and deny our humanity or will we rise to the occasion, accept the challenge, and become the heroes of this story?

Whether a test or not, I do believe that when we feel compassion and we hurt for others it's something that is placed in our hearts and minds to inspire us do something about it. It's there to act as a catalyst for change and to encourage us to use our voices, energy, and abilities to make a difference and to help those that cannot help themselves.

If you're appalled by circumstances you've read about in this book, then we need to come together and determine what we can and will do to change the system. In doing so, we must consider the kind of world that we wish to bequeath to future generations.

Do we really want our legacy to be a world that has so little respect for life forms and disastrous consequences for the long-term stability of the planet?

What will our descendants think of us in knowing that we were made aware of the vile atrocity of animal abuse yet we made the decision to disregard the feelings of other sentient beings because it was easier to pretend that such abuse wasn't happening?

What will they say when they learn that we knew of the damage to the environment caused by factory farming but we chose to ignore it so that we could continue to satiate our desire for meat and dairy products?

How will they regard our generation when they discover that we knew the truth about the secret of disease but failed to share it or use the information to provide a healthy foundation for *their* generation?

What it all comes down to is the courage to make a different decision—a decision to live up to our values.

I once thought I was doing that, and then I woke up and realized that while I was fighting for animal rights and taking a stand against cruelty toward dogs and cats, I was simultaneously taking part in the systematic destruction of other animals and our planet.

I also came to understand that believing that animals have only "one bad day" is akin to the behavior of children who still pretend to believe in Santa Claus. They go along with the fantasy, even though they're getting older and kids at school are sharing stories about their parents bringing in gifts in the middle of the night. Still, they pretend it isn't true because they think they'll have to give up the good stuff–the presents.

The decision and choice are ours. We're adults, and we make decisions every day based on our values and beliefs. We make a decision at least three times a day that will mean life or death for other living beings. In those moments of decision we also choose our quality of life. If we demand, factory farms will supply, and our health, the animals and the planet suffer the consequences. It's that simple.

At the end of the day, if we claim to love animals, we must take action. Love without action is useless. Love may be a feeling, but it's also a verb. Therefore, in order for the word love to mean anything, it requires action.

I also know that there are many people out there who desperately need the information I've shared in this book, and the majority of traditional physicians know nothing about the protein-disease connection because they're not being taught any of this in medical school, so it's up to you and me to spread the word.

I'm sure we all feel pain for those who have lost loved ones to reversible and preventable diseases because they simply didn't know the truth, and we may all cry for the animals already sacrificed for no good reason, but through our tears, and even when it feels as if our hearts are being ripped from our chest, we must believe!

We must believe that there are more good, righteous, and compassionate people than not. Then we must go and find them.

We must believe that people would care more if they only knew more. Then we must go out and educate them.

We must believe that a decision made out of irrational fear is always the wrong decision and that most people fear change due to uncertainty. Then we must go out and let them know that they're not alone and that there's nothing to fear.

I believe that there is an awakening that's taking place on our planet. I have seen it and felt it. There's an unrest that is palpable at this time in history. Human beings are waking up and realizing that they are not the *only* beings that matter. They're also waking up and realizing that they've been lied to and that they *can* control their health and the future direction of human existence.

So I call on you as an awakened soul, to take action.

I call on you to stand with those who sacrifice everything for the greater good and to answer a calling that your heart can't ignore any longer.

Together we can follow in the footsteps of the visionaries who predicted these changes and challenges years ago. We can answer the call of those who have been banging on the door and ringing the bell, trying to wake us from our slumber and warn us that our house is on fire.

> *"I am only one, but still I am one.*
> *I cannot do everything, but still I can do something.*
> *I will not refuse to do the something I can do."*
>
> ~Helen Keller

The future of our children and our children's children hang in the balance. It's not too late though. You and I can do something about it, and in the end you'll look and feel younger and have the peace of mind of knowing that you're doing everything you can to protect yourself and your loved ones from disease and disability.

You'll also know that you're making positive changes so you won't burden your loved ones as you age. You'll be mobile, disease-free, and fully functional, both physically and mentally, every day of your life. What better gift could you give not only to yourself but also to everyone you love and care about?

Your life can and will change for the better, in every possible way, if you allow this information to move you to action and make a new choice.

And if you ever question whether one person can make a difference or not, just think about Rosa Parks, Martin Luther King Jr, Mahatma Ghandi, Mother Theresa, and others who changed the world forever and will never be forgotten for their contributions to humanity.

So stand with me, and all of the other warriors for people, animals, and the planet, and help spread the word about the secret cause of disease!

About the Author

Gina Bonanno-Lemos is a Holistic Health Coach specializing in vegan nutrition practices for optimum wellness, having received her training at the Institute for Integrative Nutrition and the Vegetarian Health Institute. Gina uses her personal experience, love of food, and formal education to help men and women transition to a plant-based way of life, in the most healthful and delicious way possible.

Gina is passionate about the power of natural healing through proper nutrition, adequate rest, spirituality, and by turning past traumas into triumphs. She is also an outspoken advocate for the protection of women, children, and animals, and believes in fighting for compassion and equality for all living beings and using her voice to protect our natural resources.

When she's not cooking, advocating, or writing, you can find Gina spending time with her family, including her husband, four children, and three dogs, in Southern California.

Work With Gina Bonanno-Lemos

Looking for someone to help you get your mojo back, lose weight, and prevent disease?

As a dual Certified Integrative Nutrition Health Coach and Vegan Master, Gina works with people to not only improve and modify lifestyle and eating habits, but to help them create calm, joy, and peace in their life.

Together, you'll figure out if food is really at the core of your health issues, because as Gina likes to say, "sometimes it's not what you're eating, but what's eating you, that's the problem."

Visit the "Contact Me" page of www.360HealthConnection.com and complete the form or send a direct email to Gina@360HealthConnection.com.

Hire Gina Bonanno-Lemos to Speak at Your Next Event!

Gina has been speaking publicly and as an activist for ten years, and is an expert in the field of plant based nutrition and holistic health practices. She has created presentations which offer an overview of the material contained in this book, and can also modify her existing presentations or create entirely new presentations to match your specific theme and audience.

Visit the "Contact Me" page of www.360HealthConnection. com and complete the form or send a direct email to Gina@360HealthConnection.com.

References

Introduction

1. "Genes and Human Disease." WHO. Accessed February 11, 2016. http://www.who.int/genomics/public/geneticdiseases/en/index3.html.

2. "Genetic Testing for Hereditary Cancer Syndromes." National Cancer Institute. Accessed February 11, 2016. http://www.cancer.gov/about-cancer/causes-prevention/genetics/genetic-testing-fact-sheet.

3. Anand, Preetha, Ajaikumar B. Kunnumakara, Chitra Sundaram, Kuzhuvelil B. Harikumar, Sheeja T. Tharakan, Oiki S. Lai, Bokyung Sung, and Bharat B. Aggarwal. "Cancer Is a Preventable Disease That Requires Major Lifestyle Changes." Pharmaceutical Research. September 25, 2008. http://www.ncbi.nlm. nih.gov/pmc/articles/PMC2515569/.

What You Don't Know

1. "Farm Sanctuary." Farm Sanctuary. Accessed February 11, 2016. http://www.farmsanctuary.org/learn/factory-farming/.

2. http://www.occupyforanimals.net/animal-kill-counter.html

3. "More Than 150 Billion Animals Slaughtered Every Year." The Animal Kill Counter. Accessed February 11, 2016. http://www. adaptt.org/killcounter.html.

4. Gilam, Carey. "Retired USDA Inspectors Share Concerns About HIMP Project | Food Safety News." Food Safety News. November 16, 2015. Accessed February 11, 2016. http://www.foodsafetynews. com/2015/11/retired-usda-inspectors-share-food-safety-concerns-about-himp-project/#.Vrzy11KMQpl.

5. "Inspectors Warn Against USDA's High-Speed Hog Inspection Program." Inspectors Warn Against USDA's High-Speed Hog Inspection Program. January 30, 2015. Accessed February 11, 2016. https://www.whistleblower.org/blog/052130-inspectors-warn-against-usda's-high-speed-hog-inspection-program.

6. "Factory Farm 360 Tour." Factory Farm 360 Tour. Accessed February 11, 2016.http://factoryfarm360.org/.

7. "Continuing Problems in the USDA's Enforcement of the Humane Methods of Slaughter Act - United States House Committee on Oversight and Government Reform." United States House Committee on Oversight and Government Reform. Accessed February 11, 2016. https://oversight.house.gov/hearing/continuing-problems-in-the-usdas-enforcement-of-the-humane-methods-of-slaughter-act/.

8. "Health Management: Feedlot or Grain Bloat." Health Management: Feedlot or Grain Bloat. September 2000. Accessed February 11, 2016. http://www1.agric.gov.ab.ca/$department/deptdocs.nsf/all/beef11732.

9. Pollan, Michael. In Defense of Food: An Eater's Manifesto. New York: Penguin Press, 2008.

10. "WATCH: Undercover Investigations Expose Animal Abusers." Mercy For Animals. Accessed February 11, 2016. http://www.mercyforanimals.org/investigations.

11. Solotaroff, Paul. "Animal Cruelty Is the Price We Pay for Cheap Meat | Rolling Stone." Rolling Stone Magazine. December 10, 2013. Accessed February 11, 2016. http://www.rollingstone.com/feature/belly-beast-meat-factory-farms-animal-activists.

12. "Taking Ag-Gag to Court - Animal Legal Defense Fund." Animal Legal Defense Fund Taking AgGag to Court Comments. January 26, 2016. Accessed February 11, 2016. http://aldf.org/cases-campaigns/features/taking-ag-gag-to-court/.

13. Zelman, Joanna. "Westland/Hallmark Meat Settlement Reached After Major Meat Recall." The Huffington Post. January 16, 2013. http://www.huffingtonpost.com/2012/11/16/westland-hallmark-meat-settlement-hsus_n_2145911.html.

All My Fault

1. Joy, Melanie. "BEYOND CARNISM." Home. Accessed February 12, 2016. http://www.carnism.org/.

REFERENCES

World Destruction

1. "Ractopamine Fact Sheet Lean Meat Equals Mean Meat." Center For Food Safety. February 2013. www.centerforfoodsafety.org.

2. Rosenberg, Martha. "Ractopamine: The Meat Additive on Your Plate That's Banned Almost Everywhere But America - Cornucopia Institute." Cornucopia Institute. October 31, 2013. Accessed February 12, 2016. http://www.cornucopia.org/2013/10/ractopamine-meat-additive-plate-thats-banned-almost-everywhere-america/?utm_so.

3. Huffstutter, PJ, and Tom Polansek. "Special Report: Lost Hooves, Dead Cattle before Merck Halted Zilmax Sales." Reuters. December 31, 2013. http://www.reuters.com/article/us-zilmax-merck-cattle-special-report-idUSBRE9BT0NV20131231.

4. United States of America. Adverse Effects of Zilpaterol Administration in Horses: Three Cases. By Sarah A. Wagner, Michelle S. Mostrom, Carolyn J. Hammer, Jennifer F. Thorson, and David J. Smith. 2008. http://naldc.nal.usda.gov/download/16548/PDF.

5. Stachel, C. S., W. Radeck, and P. Gowik. "Zilpaterol—a New Focus of Concern in Residue Analysis ⊠." Zilpaterol-a New Focus of Concern in Residue Analysis. September 23, 2003. http://www.sciencedirect.com/science/article/pii/S0003267003008638.

6. Shelver, W. L., and D. J. Smith. "Tissue Residues and Urinary Excretion of Zilpaterol in Sheep Treated for 10 Days with Dietary Zilpaterol." National Center for Biotechnology Information. June 14, 2006. http://www.ncbi.nlm.nih.gov/pubmed/16756341.

7. "Food, Farm Animals, and Drugs." Antibiotic Resistance. Accessed February 12, 2016. http://www.nrdc.org/food/saving-antibiotics.asp.

8. Centers for Disease Control and Prevention. 2015. Accessed February 12, 2016. http://www.cdc.gov/drugresistance/.

9. "Antibiotic Resistance." World Health Organization. October 2015. Accessed February 12, 2016. http://www.who.int/mediacentre/factsheets/antibiotic-resistance/en/.

10. Charles, Dan. "FDA Tests Turn Up Dairy Farmers Breaking The Law On Antibiotics." NPR. March 9, 2015. Accessed February 12, 2016. http://www.npr.org/sections/thesalt/2015/03/08/391248045/fda-tests-turn-up-dairy-farmers-breaking-the-law-on-antibiotics.

11. O'Neill, Jim, and Et Al. ANTIMICROBIALS IN AGRICULTURE AND THE ENVIRONMENT:, December 2015. www.amrreview.org.

12. Chen, J., H. He, and J. Huang. "Diet Effects in Gut Microbiome and Obesity." Journal of Food Science. April 2014. http://onlinelibrary.wiley.com/doi/10.1111/1750-3841.12397/full.

13. Wlodarska, M., B. Willing, K. M. Keeney, A. Menendez, K. S. Bergstrom, N. Gill, S. L. Russell, B. A. Vallance, and B. B. Finlay. "Antibiotic Treatment Alters the Colonic Mucus Layer and Predisposes the Host to Exacerbated Citrobacter Rodentium-Induced Colitis." Infection and Immunity. February 14, 2011. http://www.ncbi.nlm.nih.gov/pmc/articles/PMC3067531/.

14. Goldsmith, Jason R., and Balfour Sartor. "The Role of Diet on Intestinal Microbiota Metabolism: Downstream Impacts on Host Immune Function and Health, and Therapeutic Implications." Journal of Gastroenterology. March 21, 2014. http://www.ncbi.nlm.nih.gov/pmc/articles/PMC4035358/#R16.

15. Nobel, Yael R., Laura M. Cox, Frances F. Kirigin, Nicholas A. Bokulich, Shingo Yamanishi, Isabel Teitler, Jennifer Chung, Jiho Sohn, Cecily M. Barber, David S. Goldfarb, Kartik Raju, Sahar Abubucker, Yanjiao Zhou, Victoria E. Ruiz, Huilin Li, Makedonka Mitreva, Alexander V. Alekseyenko, George M. Weinstock, Erica Sodergren, and Martin J. Blaser. "Metabolic and Metagenomic Outcomes from Early-life Pulsed Antibiotic Treatment." Nature.com. June 30, 2015. http://www.nature.com/ncomms/2015/150630/ncomms8486/full/ncomms8486.html.

16. Caesar, R., Fåk, F. and Bäckhed, F. (2010), Effects of gut microbiota on obesity and atherosclerosis via modulation of inflammation and lipid metabolism. Journal of Internal Medicine, 268: 320–328. doi: 10.1111/j.1365-2796.2010.02270.x

17. Polansek, Tom. "Mystery over Pig Virus Origins Contributes to Spread and Anxiety." Reuters UK. June 03, 2014. http://uk.reuters.com/article/us-pig-virus-origins-idUKKBN0EE11F20140603.

18. Na, Danny, and Tom Polansek. "U.S. Hogs Fed Pig Remains, Manure to Fend off Deadly Virus Return." Reuters India. December 14, 2015. http://in.reuters.com/article/us-usa-hogs-virus-idINKBN0TX0V520151214.

19. Emergence of plasmid-mediated colistin resistance mechanism MCR-1 in animals and human beings in China: a microbiological and

molecular biological study Liu, Yi-Yun et al. The Lancet Infectious Diseases,Volume16,Issue 2, 161-168

20. Kelland, Kate. "New "Superbug" Gene Found in Animals and People in China." Scientific American. November 19, 2015. http://www. scientificamerican.com/article/new-superbug-gene-found-in-animals-and-people-in-china/.

21. Gallagher, James. "Antibiotic Resistance: World on Cusp of 'post-antibiotic Era' - BBC News." BBC News. November 19, 2015. http://www.bbc.com/news/health-34857015.

22. United States of America. USDA. Veterinary Services Centers for Epidemiology and Animal Health. Bovine Leukosis Virus (BLV) on U.S. Dairy Operations, 2007. October 2008. https://www.aphis.usda.gov/animal_health/nahms/dairy/downloads/dairy07/Dairy07_is_BLV.pdf.

23. Buehring GC, Shen HM, Jensen HM, Jin DL, Hudes M, Block G (2015) Exposure to Bovine Leukemia Virus Is Associated with Breast Cancer: A Case-Control Study. PLoS ONE 10(9): e0134304. doi:10.1371/journal.pone.0134304

24. Buehring GC, Shen HM, Jensen HM, Choi KY, Sun D, Nuovo G. Bovine leukemia virus DNA in human breast tissue. Emerg Infect Dis [Internet]. 2014 May [date cited]. http://dx.doi.org/10.3201/eid2005.131298 DOI: 10.3201/eid2005.131298

25. Sevik, M., O. Avci, and O. B. Lnce. "An 8-year Longitudinal Sero-epidemiological Study of Bovine Leukaemia Virus (BLV) Infection in Dairy Cattle in Turkey and Analysis of Risk Factors Associated with BLV Seropositivity." National Center for Biotechnology Information. April 2015. http://www.ncbi.nlm.nih.gov/pubmed/25708566.

26. Nekoei, S., T. T. Hafshejani, A. Doosti, and F. Khamesipour. "Molecular Detection of Bovine Leukemia Virus in Peripheral Blood of Iranian Cattle, Camel and Sheep." National Center for Biotechnology Information. 2015. http://www.ncbi.nlm.nih.gov/pubmed/26812810.

27. Polat, M., S. N. Takeshima, K. Hosomichi, J. Kim, T. Miyasaka, K. Yamada, M. Arainga, T. Murakami, Y. Matsumoto, V. De La Barra Diaz, C. J. Panei, E. T. Gonzalez, M. Kanemaki, M. Onuma, G. Giovambattista, and Y. Aida. "A New Genotype of Bovine Leukemia Virus in South America Identified by NGS-based Whole Genome Sequencing and Molecular Evolutionary

Genetic Analysis." National Center for Biotechnology Information. January 12, 2016. http://www.ncbi.nlm.nih.gov/pubmed/26754835.

28. Lees, Elizabeth. "Breast Cancer Risk Linked to Virus Found in Cattle." LiveScience. September 25, 2015. http://www.livescience.com/52314-breast-cancer-risk-bovine-leukemia-virus.html.

29. Harvey, Fiona, and Andrew Wasley. "What Is the Superbug LA-MRSA CC398 and Why Is It Spreading on Farms?" The Guardian. June 18, 2015. http://www.theguardian.com/society/2015/jun/18/what-is-the-superbug-la-mrsa-cc398-and-why-is-it-spreading-on-farms.

30. Smith TC (2015) Livestock-Associated Staphylococcus aureus: The United States Experience. PLoS Pathog 11(2): e1004564. doi:10.1371/journal.ppat.1004564

31. O'Brien AM, Hanson BM, Farina SA, Wu JY, Simmering JE, Wardyn SE, et al. (2012) MRSA in Conventional and Alternative Retail Pork Products. PLoS ONE 7(1): e30092. doi:10.1371/journal.pone.0030092

32. "CANCER." Www.fda.gov. 2010. http://www.fda.gov/downloads/AdvisoryCommittees/CommitteesMeetingMaterials/TobaccoProductsScientificAdvisoryCommittee/UCM215717.pdf.

33. Silbergeld, E. K., and K. Nachman. "The Environmental and Public Health Risks Associated with Arsenical Use in Animal Feeds." National Center for Biotechnology Information. October 2008. http://www.ncbi.nlm.nih.gov/pubmed/18991934.

34. Greger, Michael, MD. "Dr. Oz, Apple Juice, and Arsenic: Chicken May Have 10 times More | NutritionFacts.org." NutritionFactsorg. September 19, 2011. http://nutritionfacts.org/2011/09/19/dr-oz-apple-juice-and-arsenic-chicken-may-have-10-times-more/.

35. Institute of Medicine (US) Committee on Curriculum Development in Environmental Medicine; Pope AM, Rall DP, editors. Environmental Medicine: Integrating a Missing Element into Medical Education. Washington (DC): National Academies Press (US); 1995. C, Case Studies in Environmental Medicine. Available from: http://www.ncbi.nlm.nih.gov/books/NBK231980/

36. Lasky, Tamar, Wenyu Sun, Abdel Kadry, and Michael K. Hoffman. "Mean Total Arsenic Concentrations in Chicken 1989–2000 and Estimated Exposures for Consumers of Chicken." January 2004. http://www.ncbi.nlm.

nih.gov/pmc/articles/PMC1241791/pdf/ehp0112-000018.pdf.

37. "Arsenic Is In Rice - Should You Worry?" EWG's Food Scores. Accessed February 18, 2016. http://www.ewg.org/foodscores/content/arsenic-contamination-in-rice.

38. Spiegel, Alison. "Chicken More Popular Than Beef In U.S. For First Time In 100 Years." The Huffington Post. January 23, 2014. http://www.huffingtonpost.com/2014/01/02/chicken-vs-beef_n_4525366.html.

39. "FDA to Withdraw Approval for Arsenic-Based Drug Used in Poultry | Food Safety News." Food Safety News. April 01, 2015. http://www.foodsafetynews.com/2015/04/fda-to-withdraw-approval-for-arsenic-based-drug-used-in-poultry/#.VsUd--aMQpl.

40. Nachman, Keeve E., Patrick A. Baron, Georg Raber, Kevin A. Francesconi, Ana Navas-Acien, and David C. Love. "EHP – Roxarsone, Inorganic Arsenic, and Other Arsenic Species in Chicken: A U.S.-Based Market Basket Sample." Environmental Health Perspectives. July 2013. http://ehp.niehs.nih.gov/1206245/.

41. "Center for Food Safety | News Room | FDA to Withdraw Approvals of Arsenic in Animal Feed." Center for Food Safety. October 1, 2013. http://www.centerforfoodsafety.org/press-releases/2620/fda-to-withdraw-approvals-of-arsenic-in-animal-feed.

42. "Center for Food Safety FOIA Complaint." 2013. http://www.centerforfoodsafety.org/files/racto_foia_complaint_final_86742.pdf.

43. "Center for Food Safety | News Room | FDA Withdraws Last Remaining Arsenic-based Animal Drug." Center for Food Safety. April 1, 2015. http://www.centerforfoodsafety.org/press-releases/3829/fda-withdraws-last-remaining-arsenic-based-animal-drug.

Weird Science

1. Smith, Jeffrey M. Genetic Roulette: The Documented Health Risks of Genetically Engineered Foods. Fairfield, IA: Yes! Books, 2007.

2. Smith, Jeffrey M. Seeds of Deception: Exposing Industry and Government Lies about the Safety of the Genetically Engineered Foods You're Eating. Fairfield, IA: Yes Books, 2003.

3. Druker, Steven M. Altered Genes, Twisted Truth::b How the Venture

to Genetically Engineer Our Food Has Subverted Science, Corrupted Government, and Systematically Deceived the Public. 1st ed. Clear River Press.

4. Gassmann AJ, Petzold-Maxwell JL, Keweshan RS, Dunbar MW (2011) Field-Evolved Resistance to Bt Maize by Western Corn Rootworm. PLoS ONE 6(7): e22629. doi:10.1371/journal.pone.0022629

5. Koebler, Jason. "Herbicide-Resistant 'Super Weeds' Increasingly Plaguing Farmers." US News. October 19, 2012. http://www.usnews.com/news/articles/2012/10/19/herbicide-resistant-super-weeds-increasingly-plaguing-farmers.

6. Heap, I. (2014), Global perspective of herbicide-resistant weeds. Pest. Manag. Sci., 70: 1306–1315. doi: 10.1002/ps.3696

7. "IARC Monographs Volume 112: Evaluation of Five Organophosphate Insecticides and Herbicides." 112 (March 20, 2015). https://www.iarc.fr/en/media-centre/iarcnews/pdf/MonographVolume112.pdf.

8. Seneff, S. , Swanson, N. and Li, C. (2015) Aluminum and Glyphosate Can Synergistically Induce Pineal Gland Pathology: Connection to Gut Dysbiosis and Neurological Disease. Agricultural Sciences, 6, 42-70. doi: 10.4236/as.2015.61005.

9. Mesnage, R., N. Defarge, J. Spiroux De Vendômois, and G. E. Seralini. "Potential Toxic Effects of Glyphosate and Its Commercial Formulations below Regulatory Limits." Potential Toxic Effects of Glyphosate and Its Commercial Formulations below Regulatory Limits. October 2015. http://www.sciencedirect.com/science/article/pii/S027869151530034X.

10. Sirinathsinghji, Eva, MD, Mae-Wan Ho, MD, and Et Al. "Banishing Glyphosate." Institute of Science in Society. September 2015. http://www.i-sis.org.uk/Banishing_Glyphosate.pdf.

11. Samsel, Anthony, and Stephanie Seneff. "Glyphosate Toxicity: Pathways to Modern Diseases." Mercola.com. December 15, 2015. http://articles.mercola.com/sites/articles/archive/2015/12/15/glyphosate-modern-diseases-pathway.aspx?e_cid=20151215Z1_DNL_art_2.

12. Kurenbach B, Marjoshi D, Amábile-Cuevas CF, Ferguson GC, Godsoe W, Gibson P, Heinemann JA. 2015. Sublethal

REFERENCES

exposure to commercial formulations of the herbicides dicamba, 2,4-dichlorophenoxyacetic acid, and glyphosate cause changes in antibiotic susceptibility in Escherichia coli and Salmonella enterica serovar Typhimurium. mBio 6(2):e00009-15. doi:10.1128/mBio.00009-15.

13. "GMOs, Glyphosate and Mitochondrial Dysfunction." Institute for Responsible Technology. December 9, 2015. http://responsibletechnology.org/gmos-and-mitochondrial-dysfunction/.

14. Hoy J, Swanson N, Seneff S (2015) The High Cost of Pesticides: Human and Animal Diseases. Poult Fish Wildl Sci 3:132. doi:10.4172/2375-446X.1000132

15. Ho, Mae-Wan, MD, and Joe Cummins, PhD. "Glyphosate Toxic & Roundup Worse." Institute of Science in Society. July 3, 2005. http://www.i-sis.org.uk/GTARW.php.

16. Mesnage, Robin, Nicolas Defarge, Joël Spiroux De Vendômois, and Gilles-Eric Séralini. "Major Pesticides Are More Toxic to Human Cells Than Their Declared Active Principles." BioMed Research International. February 26, 2014. https://www.ncbi.nlm.nih.gov/pmc/articles/PMC3955666/.

17. Ho, Mae-Wan, MD, and Brett Cherry. "Death by Multiple Poisoning, Glyphosate and Roundup." Institute of Science in Society. November 2, 2009. http://www.i-sis.org.uk/DMPGR.php.

18. Benachour, N., and G. E. Seralini. "Glyphosate Formulations Induce Apoptosis and Necrosis in Human Umbilical, Embryonic, and Placental Cells." National Center for Biotechnology Information. January 22, 2009. http://www.ncbi.nlm.nih.gov/pubmed/19105591.

19. López-Armada, M. J., R. R. Riveiro-Naveira, C. Vaamonde-García, and M. N. Valcárcel-Ares. "Mitochondrial Dysfunction and the Inflammatory Response." National Center for Biotechnology Information. March 13, 2013. http://www.ncbi.nlm.nih.gov/pubmed/23333405.

20. Lopez, J., and SW G. Tait. "Mitochondrial Apoptosis: Killing Cancer Using the Enemy within." Nature.com. March 5, 2015. http://www.nature.com/bjc/journal/v112/n6/full/bjc201585a.html.

21. Kim, Jung-whan, and Chi V. Dang. "Cancer's Molecular Sweet Tooth

and the Warburg Effect." Cancer Research. September 15, 2006. http://cancerres.aacrjournals.org/content/66/18/8927.full.

22. Christofferson, Travis. Tripping over the Truth: The Metabolic Theory of Cancer. Create Space Independent Publishing Platform, 2014.

23. Frye, Richard E., and Daniel A. Rossignol. "Mitochondrial Dysfunction Can Connect the Diverse Medical Symptoms Associated with Autism Spectrum Disorders." Pediatric Research. May 1, 2012. http://www.ncbi.nlm.nih.gov/pmc/articles/PMC3179978/.

24. Madamanchi, Nageswara R., and Marschall S. Runge. "Mitochondrial Dysfunction in Atherosclerosis." Mitochondrial Dysfunction in Atherosclerosis. 2007. doi:10.1161/01. RES.0000258450.44413.96.

25. Davi, Alyssa. "Does Mitochondrial Dysfunction Finally Connect the Diverse Medical Symptoms We Now See in Children With Various Health Problems?" Epidemic Answers. October 22, 2013. http://www.epidemicanswers.org/does-mitochondrial-dysfunction-finally-connect-the-diverse-medical-symptoms-we-now-see-in-children-with-various-health-problems/.

26. Cordero, M. D., M. De Miguel, I. Carmona-Lopez, P. Bonal, F. Campa, and A. M. Moreno-Fernandez. "Oxidative Stress and Mitochondrial Dysfunction in Fibromyalgia." National Center for Biotechnology Information. 2010. http://www.ncbi.nlm.nih.gov/pubmed/20424583.

27. "Mitochondrial Defects Are a Central Factor in Human Health and Disease." - The United Mitochondrial Disease Foundation. Accessed February 19, 2016. http://www.umdf.org/site/pp.aspx?c=8qKOJ0MvF7LUG.

28. University of California - Davis Health System. "Children with autism have mitochondrial dysfunction, study finds." ScienceDaily. ScienceDaily, 30 November 2010. <www.sciencedaily.com/releases/2010/11/101130161521.htm>

29. Scaglia, Fernando. "THE ROLE OF MITOCHONDRIAL DYSFUNCTION IN PSYCHIATRIC DISEASE." 2010. http://isites.harvard.edu/fs/docs/icb.topic889975.files/April 4th/Additional readings APril 4th/Scaglia 2010.pdf.

30. Aris, A., and S. Leblanc. "Result Filters." National Center for Biotechnology Information. May 31, 2011. http://www.ncbi.nlm.nih.gov/pubmed/21338670.

31. Latham, Jonathan R., PhD. "Growing Doubt: A Scientist's Experience of GMOs." Independent Science News Food Health and Agriculture Bioscience News. August 31, 2015. http://www.independentsciencenews.org/health/growing-doubt-a-scientists-experience-of-gmos/.

32. Podevin, N., and P. Du Jardin. "Possible Consequences of the Overlap between the CaMV 35S Promoter Regions in Plant Transformation Vectors Used and the Viral Gene VI in Transgenic Plants." National Center for Biotechnology Information. December 2012. http://www.ncbi.nlm.nih.gov/pubmed/22892689.

33. Latham, Jonathan, PhD, and Alison Wilson, PhD. "Is the Hidden Viral Gene Safe? GMO Regulators Fail to Convince." Independent Science News. February 27, 2013. https://www.independentsciencenews.org/health/gmo-regulators-hidden-viral-gene-vi-regulators-fail/.

34. Ho, Mae-Wan. "Potentially Dangerous Virus Gene Hidden in Commercial GM Crops." Institute of Science in Society. January 28, 2013. http://www.i-sis.org.uk/Potentially_Dangerous_Virus_Gene_in_GM_Crops.php.

35. "The Cauliflower Mosaic Virus Promoter in GM Crops: Should We Worry?" GMWatch. January 1, 2015. http://www.gmwatch.org/news/archive/2014/87-news/archive/2015/15838-the-cauliflower-mosaic-virus-promoter-in-gm-crops-should-we-worry.

36. Hanaa A. S. Oraby, Mahrousa M. H. Kandil, Amal A. M. Hassan and Hayam A. Al-Sharawi. "Addressing the issue of horizontal gene transfer from a diet containing genetically modified components into rat tissues." African Journal of Biotechnology 13, no. 48 (2014): 4410-4418.

37. Campbell, Andrew W. "Autoimmunity and the Gut." National Institutes of Health. Hindawi Publishing Corporation, 13 May 2014. Web. 10.1155/2014/152428

38. Lodish, Harvey. "Transport across Epithelia." National Institutes of

Health. U.S. National Library of Medicine. Web. 21 Feb. 2016.

39. Samsel, Anthony, and Stephanie Seneff. "Glyphosate, Pathways to Modern '] Diseases II: Celiac Sprue and Gluten Intolerance." Interdisciplinary Toxicology. December 2013. http://www.ncbi.nlm. nih.gov/pmc/articles/PMC3945755/.

40. Smith, Jeffrey, and Zach Bush, MD. "Jeffrey Smith Interviews Zach Bush on Glyphosate & the Nervous System - Restore." Restore. February 17, 2016. http://restore4life.com/jeffrey-smith-interviews-zach-bush-on-glyphosate-the-nervous-system/?mc_cid=ed547fcd53.

41. Blum, Susan S., and Michele Bender. The Immune System Recovery Plan: A Doctor's 4-step Program to Treat Autoimmune Disease. 1st ed. Scribner, 2013.

42. Carmen, Judy A., Howard R. Vileger, Larry J. Ver Steeg, Verlyn E. Sneller, Garth W. Robinson, Catherine A. Clinch-Jones, Julie L. Haynes, and John W. Edwards. "A Long-term Toxicology Study on Pigs Fed a Combined Genetically Modified (GM) Soy and GM Maize Diet." Gmojudycarman.org. 2013. http://gmojudycarman.org/wp-content/uploads/2013/06/The-Full-Paper.pdf.

43. "Glyphosate Research Papers Compiled By Dr Alex Vasquez and Dr Eva Sirinathsinghji." Institute of Science in Society. Accessed February 22, 2016. http://www.i-sis.org.uk/pdf/Glyphosate_research_papers_compiled_by_Dr_Alex_Vasquez_and_Dr_Eva_Sirinathsinghji.pdf.

44. "OCA Addresses Organic Standards Issues at Spring NOSB Meeting." Organic Consumers Association. April 27, 2015. https://www.organicconsumers.org/press/oca-addresses-organic-standards-issues-spring-nosb-meeting.

45. Endres, A. Bryan, and Stephanie B. Johnson. "Distinguishing Marketing Claims for Grass-fed, Organic, and Pasture-raised Livestock." Illinois State Bar Association. January 2010. https://www.isba.org/sections/animallaw/newsletter/2010/01/distinguishingmarketingclaimsforgrassfedorganicandpa.

46. Philpott, Tom. "Wait, We Inject Antibiotics into Organic Chicken Eggs?!" Mother Jones. January 15, 2014. http://www.motherjones.com/tom-philpott/2014/01/organic-chicken-and-egg-antibiotics-edition.

47. Greenaway, Twilight, and Adrien Schless-Meier. "Just Because Your Chicken Is Organic Doesn't Mean It Was Raised Humanely." Just Because Your Chicken Is Organic Doesn't Mean It Was Raised Humanely. April 23, 2015. https://www.organicconsumers.org/news/just-because-your-chicken-organic-doesnt-mean-it-was-raised-humanely.

48. "The Organic and 'Free-Range' Myth." PETA. Accessed February 22, 2016. http://www.peta.org/issues/animals-used-for-food/free-range-organic-meat-myth/.

49. "Animals Used for Free-Range and Organic Meat." PETA. Accessed February 22, 2016. http://www.peta.org/issues/animals-used-for-food/organic-free-range-meat/.

50. "Free-Range and Organic Meat, Eggs, and Dairy Products: Conning Consumers?" PETA. Accessed February 22, 2016. http://www.peta.org/issues/animals-used-for-food/animals-used-food-factsheets/free-range-organic-meat-eggs-dairy-products-conning-consumers/.

51. "The Truth Behind "Humane" Meat, Milk, And Eggs." Farm Sanctuary. April 21, 2009. http://www.farmsanctuary.org/wp-content/uploads/2012/03/Truth-Behind-Humane-FINAL-4-21-09.pdf.

52. Guarino, Ben. "Killing Wolves To Protect Farm Animals Backfires." The Dodo. December 4, 2014. https://www.thedodo.com/wolf-hunts-backfire-856736320.html.

53. "Minnesota Farmers Face a 'perfect Storm' Because of Wolf Ruling." Star Tribune. February 21, 2015. http://www.startribune.com/minnesota-farmers-face-a-perfect-storm-because-of-wolf-ruling/293284661/.

You Be Illin'

1. Mozaffarian, Dariush, Emelia J. Benjamin, Alan S. Go, Donna K. Arnett, Michael J. Blaha, Mary Cushman, Sandeep R. Das, Sarah De Ferranti, Jean-Pierre Després, Heather J. Fullerton, Virginia J. Howard, Mark D. Huffman, Carmen R. Isasi, Monik C. Jiménez, Suzanne E. Judd, Brett M. Kissela, Judith H. Lichtman, Lynda D. Lisabeth, Simin Liu, Rachel H. Mackey, David J. Magid, Darren K. Mcguire, Emile R. Mohler, Claudia S. Moy, Paul Muntner,

Michael E. Mussolino, Khurram Nasir, Robert W. Neumar, Graham Nichol, Latha Palaniappan, Dilip K. Pandey, Mathew J. Reeves, Carlos J. Rodriguez, Wayne Rosamond, Paul D. Sorlie, Joel Stein, Amytis Towfighi, Tanya N. Turan, Salim S. Virani, Daniel Woo, Robert W. Yeh, and Melanie B. Turner. "Heart Disease and Stroke Statistics—2016 Update." Circulation, December 16, 2015. http://circ.ahajournals.org/content/early/2015/12/16/CIR.0000000000000350.full.pdf.

2. "Meat and Eggs Increase Risk for Stroke." The Physicians Committee. November 12, 2015. https://www.pcrm.org/health/medNews/meat-and-eggs-increase-risk-for-stroke.

3. Pan, A., Q. Sun, A. M. Bernstein, M. B. Schulze, J. E. Manson, M. J. Stampfer, W. C. Willett, and F. B. Hu. "Unbound MEDLINE : Red Meat Consumption and Mortality: Results from 2 Prospective Cohort Studie." Unbound MEDLINE : Red Meat Consumption and Mortality: Results from 2 Prospective Cohort Studie. April 9, 2012. http://www.unboundmedicine.com/medline/citation/22412075/Red_meat_consumption_and_mortality:_results_from_2_prospective_cohort_studies_.

4. Takata, Yumie, Xiao-Ou Shu, Yu-Tang Gao, Honglan Li, Xianglan Zhang, Jing Gao, Hui Cai, Gong Yang, Yong-Bing Xiang, and Wei Zheng. "Red Meat and Poultry Intakes and Risk of Total and Cause-Specific Mortality: Results from Cohort Studies of Chinese Adults in Shanghai." PLoS ONE 8, no. 2 (February 22, 2013). http://journals.plos.org/plosone/article?id=10.1371/journal.pone.0056963.

5. Rohrmann, S., Et Al. "Result Filters." National Center for Biotechnology Information. March 7, 2013. http://www.ncbi.nlm.nih.gov/pubmed/23497300.

6. Wiseman, M. "55 Food, Nutrition, Physical Activity, and Cancer Prevention - World Cancer Research Fund (WCRF)." American Institute for Cancer Research 48 (2012). http://www.aicr.org/assets/docs/pdf/reports/Second_Expert_Report.pdf.

7. Fung, Teresa T., R. M. Van Dam, S. E. Hankinson, M. Stampfer, W. C. Willett, and F. B. Hu. "Low-Carbohydrate Diets and All-Cause and Cause-Specific Mortality." Annals of Internal Medicine Ann Intern Med 153, no. 5 (September 07, 2010): 289. http://www.ncbi.

nlm.nih.gov/pubmed/20820038.

8. Wang, Xia, Xinying Lin, Ying Y. Ouyang, Jun Liu, Gang Zhao, An Pan, and Frank B. Hu. "Red and Processed Meat Consumption and Mortality: Dose–response Meta-analysis of Prospective Cohort Studies." Public Health Nutr. Public Health Nutrition, July 06, 2015, 1-13. http://www.ncbi.nlm.nih.gov/pubmed/26143683.

9. Tang, W.h., Z. Wang, and B.s. Levison. "Intestinal Microbial Metabolism of Phosphatidylcholine and Cardiovascular Risk." Journal of Vascular Surgery 58, no. 2 (April 25, 2013): 549. http://www.nejm.org/doi/full/10.1056/NEJMoa1109400.

10. Koeth, Robert A., Zeneng Wang, Bruce S. Levison, Jennifer A. Buffa, Elin Org, Brendan T. Sheehy, Earl B. Britt, Xiaoming Fu, Yuping Wu, Lin Li, Jonathan D. Smith, Joseph A. Didonato, Jun Chen, Hongzhe Li, Gary D. Wu, James D. Lewis, Manya Warrier, J. Mark Brown, Ronald M. Krauss, W. H Wilson Tang, Frederic D. Bushman, Aldons J. Lusis, and Stanley L. Hazen. "Intestinal Microbiota Metabolism of L-carnitine, a Nutrient in Red Meat, Promotes Atherosclerosis." Nature Medicine Nat Med 19, no. 5 (April 07, 2013): 576-85. http://www.ncbi.nlm.nih.gov/pmc/articles/PMC3650111/.

11. Tang, W. H. W., Z. Wang, D. J. Kennedy, Y. Wu, J. A. Buffa, B. Agatisa-Boyle, X. S. Li, B. S. Levison, and S. L. Hazen. "Gut Microbiota-Dependent Trimethylamine N-Oxide (TMAO) Pathway Contributes to Both Development of Renal Insufficiency and Mortality Risk in Chronic Kidney Disease." Circulation Research 116, no. 3 (January 30, 2015): 448-55. http://www.ncbi.nlm.nih.gov/pubmed/25599331.

12. Koeth, Robert A., Bruce S. Levison, Miranda K. Culley, Jennifer A. Buffa, Zeneng Wang, Jill C. Gregory, Elin Org, Yuping Wu, Lin Li, Jonathan D. Smith, W.h. Wilson Tang, Joseph A. Didonato, Aldons J. Lusis, and Stanley L. Hazen. "⊠-Butyrobetaine Is a Proatherogenic Intermediate in Gut Microbial Metabolism of L-Carnitine to TMAO." Cell Metabolism 20, no. 5 (November 4, 2014): 799-812. http://www.ncbi.nlm.nih.gov/pubmed/25440057.

13. David, Lawrence A., Corinne F. Maurice, Rachel N. Carmody, David B. Gootenberg, Julie E. Button, Benjamin E. Wolfe, Alisha V. Ling, A. Sloan Devlin, Yug Varma, Michael A. Fischbach, Sudha B.

Biddinger, Rachel J. Dutton, and Peter J. Turnbaugh. "Diet Rapidly and Reproducibly Alters the Human Gut Microbiome." Nature 505, no. 7484 (December 11, 2013): 559-63. http://www.nature.com/nature/journal/v505/n7484/full/nature12820.html.

14. Schwartz, B. G., and R. A. Kloner. "Cardiovascular Implications of Erectile Dysfunction." American Heart Association Journals 123.21 (2011). Web. <http://circ.ahajournals.org/content/123/21/e609.full>.

15. "Heart Disease." Mayo Clinic. 29 July 2014. Web.

16. "National Diabetes Statistics Report, 2014." Centers for Disease Control and Prevention. 2014. http://www.cdc.gov/diabetes/pubs/statsreport14/national-diabetes-report-web.pdf.

17. "Diabetes." World Health Organization. January 2015. http://www.who.int/mediacentre/factsheets/fs312/en/.

18. "Statistics About Diabetes." American Diabetes Association. June 10, 2014. http://www.diabetes.org/diabetes-basics/statistics/.

19. "2014 National Diabetes Statistics Report." Centers for Disease Control and Prevention. May 15, 2015. http://www.cdc.gov/diabetes/data/statistics/2014StatisticsReport.html.

20. Pan, A., Q. Sun, A. M. Bernstein, M. B. Schulze, J. E. Manson, W. C. Willett, and F. B. Hu. "Red Meat Consumption and Risk of Type 2 Diabetes: 3 Cohorts of US Adults and an Updated Meta-analysis." American Journal of Clinical Nutrition 94.4 (2011): 1088-096. Web.

21. Shaw, Jonathan. "A Diabetes Link to Meat." Harvard Magazine. February 2012. http://harvardmagazine.com/2012/01/a-diabetes-link-to-meat.

22. "Global Prevalence of Diabetes Estimates for the Year 2000 and Projections for 2030." American Diabetes Association. May 2004. http://care.diabetesjournals.org/content/27/5/1047.full.

23. Fagherazzi, Guy, Alice Vilier, Fabrice Bonnet, Martin Lajous, Beverley Balkau, Marie-Christine Boutron-Ruault, and Françoise Clavel-Chapelon. "Dietary Acid Load and Risk of Type 2 Diabetes: The E3N-EPIC Cohort Study." Diabetologia 57, no. 2 (October 14, 2013): 313-20. http://www.nutrinfo.com/biblioteca/documentos_adicionales/Fagherazzi.pdf.

24. McMacken, Michelle, MD. "7 Things That Happen When You Stop Eating Meat." Forks Over Knives. January 12, 2016. http://www. forksoverknives.com/7-things-that-happen-when-you-stop-eating-meat/.

25. Miedema, Michael D., Andrew Petrone, James Shikany, Philip Greenland, Cora Lewis, Mark Pletcher, J. Michael Gaziano, and Luc Djousse. "The Association Of Fruit And Vegetable Consumption During Early Adulthood With The Prevalence Of Coronary Artery Calcium After 20 Years Of Follow-Up: The Coronary Artery Risk Development In Young Adults (Cardia) Study." Journal of the American College of Cardiology 63, no. 12 (November 24, 2014). http://www.ncbi.nlm.nih.gov/pubmed/26503880.

26. Rumawas, Marcella E., Nicola M. Mckeown, Gail Rogers, James B. Meigs, Peter W.f. Wilson, and Paul F. Jacques. "Magnesium Intake Is Related to Improved Insulin Homeostasis in the Framingham Offspring Cohort." Journal of the American College of Nutrition 25, no. 6 (December 25, 2006): 486-92. http://www.ncbi.nlm.nih.gov/pubmed/17229895.

27. Wang, Jinsong, Gioia Persuitte, Barbara Olendzki, Nicole Wedick, Zhiying Zhang, Philip Merriam, Hua Fang, James Carmody, Gin-Fei Olendzki, and Yunsheng Ma. "Dietary Magnesium Intake Improves Insulin Resistance among Non-Diabetic Individuals with Metabolic Syndrome Participating in a Dietary Trial." Nutrients 5, no. 10 (September 27, 2013): 3910-919. http://www.mdpi.com/2072-6643/5/10/3910.

28. Hruby, A., J. B. Meigs, C. J. O'donnell, P. F. Jacques, and N. M. Mckeown. "Higher Magnesium Intake Reduces Risk of Impaired Glucose and Insulin Metabolism and Progression From Prediabetes to Diabetes in Middle-Aged Americans." Diabetes Care 37, no. 2 (October 02, 2013): 419-27. http://care.diabetesjournals.org/content/early/2013/09/23/dc13-1397.short.

29. Le, Lap, and Joan Sabaté. "Beyond Meatless, the Health Effects of Vegan Diets: Findings from the Adventist Cohorts." Nutrients 6, no. 6 (May 27, 2014): 2131-/147. http://www.ncbi.nlm.nih.gov/pmc/articles/PMC4073139/.

30. Jenkins, David JA, Cyril WC Kendall, Augustine Marchie, Alexandra

L. Jenkins, Livia SA Augustin, David S. Ludwig, Neal D. Barnard, and James W. Anderson. "The American Journal of Clinical Nutrition." Type 2 Diabetes and the Vegetarian Diet. September 2003. http://ajcn.nutrition.org/content/78/3/610S.full#ref-6.

31. Trapp, C., and S. Levin. "Preparing to Prescribe Plant-Based Diets for Diabetes Prevention and Treatment." Diabetes Spectrum 25, no. 1 (February 01, 2012): 38-44. http://spectrum.diabetesjournals.org/content/25/1/38.full.

32. Nagura, Junko, Hiroyasu Iso, Yoshiyuki Watanabe, Koutatsu Maruyama, Chigusa Date, Hideaki Toyoshima, Akio Yamamoto, Shogo Kikuchi, Akio Koizumi, Takaaki Kondo, Yasuhiko Wada, Yutaka Inaba, and Akiko Tamakoshi. "Fruit, Vegetable and Bean Intake and Mortality from Cardiovascular Disease among Japanese Men and Women: The JACC Study." BJN British Journal of Nutrition 102, no. 02 (January 13, 2009): 285. http://journals.cambridge.org/action/

33. Cassidy, A., M. Franz, and E. B. Rimm. "Dietary Flavonoid Intake and Incidence of Erectile Dysfunction." American Journal of Clinical Nutrition 103, no. 2 (January 13, 2016): 534-41. http://ajcn.nutrition.org/content/early/2016/01/06/ajcn.115.122010.abstract.

34. Barnard, Neal, Susan Levin, and Caroline Trapp. "Meat Consumption as a Risk Factor for Type 2 Diabetes." Nutrients 6, no. 2 (February 21, 2014): 897-910. http://www.ncbi.nlm.nih.gov/pmc/articles/PMC3942738/pdf/nutrients-06-00897.pdf.

35. Campbell, T. Colin, and Thomas M. Campbell. The China Study: The Most Comprehensive Study of Nutrition Ever Conducted and the Startling Implications for Diet, Weight Loss and Long-term Health. Dallas, TX: BenBella Books, 2005.

36. "IARC Monographs Evaluate Consumption of Red Meat and Processed Meat." International Agency for Research on Cancer. October 26, 2015. https://www.iarc.fr/en/media-centre/pr/2015/pdfs/pr240_E.pdf.

37. Bradbury, K.e., and T.j. Key. "The Association of Red and Processed Meat, and Dietary Fibre with Colorectal Cancer in UK Biobank." Proceedings of the Nutrition Society Proc. Nutr. Soc. 74, no. OCE5 (November 2015). 7/S0029665115003365.

REFERENCES

38. Richman, E. L., S. A. Kenfield, M. J. Stampfer, E. L. Giovannucci, S. H. Zeisel, W. C. Willett, and J. M. Chan. "Choline Intake and Risk of Lethal Prostate Cancer: Incidence and Survival." American Journal of Clinical Nutrition 96, no. 4 (September 05, 2012): 855-63. http://www.ncbi.nlm. nih.gov/pubmed/22952174.

39. Richman, E. L., S. A. Kenfield, M. J. Stampfer, E. L. Giovannucci, and J. M. Chan. "Egg, Red Meat, and Poultry Intake and Risk of Lethal Prostate Cancer in the Prostate-Specific Antigen-Era: Incidence and Survival." Cancer Prevention Research 4, no. 12 (September 19, 2011): 2110-121. http://www.ncbi.nlm.nih.gov/pubmed/21930800.

40. Zhu, Hong-Cheng, Xi Yang, Li-Ping Xu, Lian-Jun Zhao, Guang-Zhou Tao, Chi Zhang, Qin Qin, Jing Cai, Jian-Xin Ma, Wei-Dong Mao, Xi-Zhi Zhang, Hong-Yan Cheng, and Xin-Chen Sun. "Meat Consumption Is Associated with Esophageal Cancer Risk in a Meat- and Cancer-Histological-Type Dependent Manner." Dig Dis Sci Digestive Diseases and Sciences 59, no. 3 (January 07, 2014): 664-73. http://www.ncbi.nlm. nih.gov/pubmed/24395380.

41. Kim, Andre E., Abbie Lundgreen, Roger K. Wolff, Laura Fejerman, Esther M. John, Gabriela Torres-Mejía, Sue A. Ingles, Stephanie D. Boone, Avonne E. Connor, Lisa M. Hines, Kathy B. Baumgartner, Anna Giuliano, Amit D. Joshi, Martha L. Slattery, and Mariana C. Stern. "Red Meat, Poultry, and Fish Intake and Breast Cancer Risk among Hispanic and Non-Hispanic White Women: The Breast Cancer Health Disparities Study." Cancer Causes & Control Cancer Causes Control, February 22, 2016. http://www.ncbi.nlm.nih.gov/pubmed/26898200.

42. Nothlings, U., L. R. Wilkens, S. P. Murphy, J. H. Hankin, B. E. Henderson, and L. N. Kolonel. "Meat and Fat Intake as Risk Factors for Pancreatic Cancer: The Multiethnic Cohort Study." JNCI Journal of the National Cancer Institute 97, no. 19 (October 5, 2005): 1458-465. http://www.ncbi.nlm.nih.gov/pubmed/16204695?log$=activity.

43. Hooda, Jagmohan, Ajit Shah, and Li Zhang. "Heme, an Essential Nutrient from Dietary Proteins, Critically Impacts Diverse Physiological and Pathological Processes." Nutrients 6, no. 3 (March 13, 2014): 1080-102. http://www.ncbi.nlm.nih.gov/pmc/articles/PMC3967179/.

44. Bardor, Muriel, Dzung H. Nguyen, Sandra Diaz, and Ajit Varki. "Mechanism of Uptake and Incorporation of the Non-human Sialic Acid

N -Glycolylneuraminic Acid into Human Cells." Journal of Biological Chemistry J. Biol. Chem. 280, no. 6 (November 22, 2004): 4228-237. http://www.jbc.org/content/280/6/4228.full.

45. Pearce, Oliver M., PhD. "Oliver M. Pearce: Exploring the Link Between Western Diets and Cancer." Cancer Research Institute. Accessed February 25, 2016. http://www.cancerresearch.org/our-strategy-impact/people-behind-the-progress/scientists/oliver-m-pearce-exploring-the-link-between-weste.

46. Wang, B. "Molecular Mechanism Underlying Sialic Acid as an Essential Nutrient for Brain Development and Cognition." Advances in Nutrition: An International Review Journal 3, no. 3 (May 01, 2012). http:/advances.nutrition.org/content/3/3/465S.full.

47. Hedlund, M., V. Padler-Karavani, N. M. Varki, and A. Varki. "Evidence for a Human-specific Mechanism for Diet and Antibody-mediated Inflammation in Carcinoma Progression." Proceedings of the National Academy of Sciences 105, no. 48 (October 8, 2008): 18936-8941. http://www.pnas.org/content/105/48/18936.full.pdf.

48. Samraj, Annie N., Oliver M. T. Pearce, Heinz Läubli, Alyssa N. Crittenden, Anne K. Bergfeld, Kalyan Banda, Christopher J. Gregg, Andrea E. Bingman, Patrick Secrest, Sandra L. Diaz, Nissi M. Varki, and Ajit Varki. "A Red Meat-derived Glycan Promotes Inflammation and Cancer Progression." Proceedings of the National Academy of Sciences Proc Natl Acad Sci USA 112, no. 2 (November 25, 2014): 542-47. http://www.pnas.org/content/112/2/542.abstract.

49. Tangvoranuntakul, P., P. Gagneux, S. Diaz, M. Bardor, N. Varki, A. Varki, and E. Muchmore. "Human Uptake and Incorporation of an Immunogenic Nonhuman Dietary Sialic Acid." Proceedings of the National Academy of Sciences 100, no. 21 (October 01, 2003): 12045-2050. http://www.ncbi.nlm.nih.gov/pmc/articles/PMC218710/.

50. Samraj, Annie N., Heinz Läubli, Nissi Varki, and Ajit Varki. "Involvement of a Non-Human Sialic Acid in Human Cancer." Front. Oncol. Frontiers in Oncology 4 (February 19, 2014). http://journal.frontiersin.org/article/10.3389/fonc.2014.00033/full.

51. Hart, B. A. 't. "Why Does Multiple Sclerosis Only Affect Human Primates?" Multiple Sclerosis Journal, June 25, 2015. http://www.ncbi.nlm.nih.gov/pubmed/26540733.

52. Kobayashi, Lindsay. "Red Meat and Cancer: The Biological Evidence | Public Health." Public Health. 17 Nov. 2014. Web.

53. Eleftheriou, Phaedra, Stavros Kynigopoulos, Alexandra Giovou, Alexandra Mazmanidi, John Yovos, Petros Skepastianos, Eleni Vagdatli, Christos Petrou, Dafni Papara, and Maria Efterpiou. "Prevalence of Anti-Neu5Gc Antibodies in Patients with Hypothyroidism." BioMed Research International 2014 (June 9, 2014): 1-9. http://www.ncbi.nlm.nih.gov/pmc/articles/PMC4070528/.

54. Bogovski, P., and S. Bogovski. "Special Report Animal Species in Whichn-nitroso Compounds Induce Cancer." International Journal of Cancer Int. J. Cancer 27.4 (1981): 471-74. Web.

55. Bastide, N. M., F. H. F. Pierre, and D. E. Corpet. "Heme Iron from Meat and Risk of Colorectal Cancer: A Meta-analysis and a Review of the Mechanisms Involved." Cancer Prevention Research 4.2 (2011): 177-84. Web. <http://cancerpreventionresearch.aacrjournals.org/content/4/2/177.long>.

56. "Red and Processed Meat Products: No Safe Amount." Physicians Committee for Responsible Medicine. Web. 26 Feb. 2016. <http://www.pcrm.org/sites/default/files/pdfs/dropthedog/Red and processed meat fact sheet.pdf>.

57. "Table 4. Food Sources of Arachidonic Acid (PFA 20:4), Listed in Descending Order by Percentages of Their Contribution to Intake, Based on Data from the National Health and Nutrition Examination Survey 2005-2006." Food Sources of Arachidonic Acid (PFA 20:4), Listed in Descending Order by Percentages of Their Contribution to Intake, Based on Data from the National Health and Nutrition Examination Survey 2005-2006. October 18, 2013. http://appliedresearch.cancer.gov/diet/foodsources/fatty_acids/table4.html.

58. Li, Duo, Alice Ng, Neil J. Mann, and Andrew J. Sinclair. "Contribution of Meat Fat to Dietary Arachidonic Acid." Lipids 33, no. 4 (August 1998): 437-40. http://www.ncbi.nlm.nih.gov/pubmed/9590632.

59. Zheng, Wei, and Sang-Ah Lee. "Well-Done Meat Intake, Heterocyclic Amine Exposure, and Cancer Risk." Nutrition and Cancer 61, no. 4 (2009): 437-46. http://www.ncbi.nlm.nih.gov/pmc/articles/PMC2769029/.

60. "Chemicals in Meat Cooked at High Temperatures and Cancer Risk." National Cancer Institute. Accessed February 27, 2016. http://www.cancer.gov/about-cancer/causes-prevention/risk/diet/cooked-meats-fact-sheet.

61. Busch, Christian, Markus Burkard, Christian Leischner, Ulrich M. Lauer, Jan Frank, and Sascha Venturelli. "Epigenetic Activities of Flavonoids in the Prevention and Treatment of Cancer." Clinical Epigenetics Clin Epigenet 7, no. 1 (July 10, 2015). http://www.ncbi.nlm.nih.gov/pmc/articles/PMC4497414/.

62. Shankar, Sharmila, Dhruv Kumar, and Rakesh K. Srivastava. "Epigenetic Modifications by Dietary Phytochemicals: Implications for Personalized Nutrition." Pharmacology & Therapeutics 138, no. 1 (April 2013): 1-17. http://www.ncbi.nlm.nih.gov/pmc/articles/PMC4153856/.

63. Ong, Thomas Prates, Fernando Salvador Moreno, and Sharon Ann Ross. "Targeting the Epigenome with Bioactive Food Components for Cancer Prevention." Journal of Nutrigenetics and Nutrigenomics J Nutrigenet Nutrigenomics 4, no. 5 (February 22, 2012): 275-92. http://www.ncbi.nlm.nih.gov/pmc/articles/PMC3388269/.

64. Koyyalamudi, Sundar Rao, Sang-Chul Jeong, Chi-Hyun Song, Kai Yip Cho, and Gerald Pang. "Vitamin D2 Formation and Bioavailability from Agaricus Bisporus ?Button Mushrooms Treated with Ultraviolet Irradiation." J. Agric. Food Chem. Journal of Agricultural and Food Chemistry 57.8 (2009): 3351-355. Web. <http://www.ncbi.nlm.nih.gov/pubmed/19281276>.

65. Haritan, Adam. "5 Unique Health Benefits Of Morel Mushrooms." Wild Foodism. 2014. http://wildfoodism.com/2014/04/02/5-unique-health-benefits-of-morel-mushrooms/.

66. Ornish, Dean, Jue Lin, June M. Chan, Elissa Epel, Colleen Kemp, Gerdi Weidner, Ruth Marlin, Steven J. Frenda, Mark Jesus M Magbanua, Jennifer Daubenmier, Ivette Estay, Nancy K. Hills, Nita Chainani-Wu, Peter R. Carroll, and Elizabeth H. Blackburn. "Effect of Comprehensive Lifestyle Changes on Telomerase Activity and Telomere Length in Men with Biopsy-proven Low-risk Prostate Cancer: 5-year Follow-up of a Descriptive Pilot Study." The Lancet Oncology 14, no. 11 (October 2013): 1112-120. http://www.ncbi.nlm.nih.gov/pubmed/24051140.

67. Kerstetter, Jane E., Kimberly O. O'Brien, Donna M. Caseria, Diane E. Wall, and Karl L. Insogna. "The Impact of Dietary Protein on Calcium

Absorption and Kinetic Measures of Bone Turnover in Women." The Journal of Clinical Endocrinology & Metabolism 90, no. 1 (February 5, 2004): 26-31. http://press.endocrine.org/doi/10.1210/jc.2004-0179?url_ver=Z39.88-2003&rfr_id=ori:rid:crossref.org&rfr_dat=cr_pub=pubmed&.

68. Cao, J. J., L. K. Johnson, and J. R. Hunt. "A Diet High in Meat Protein and Potential Renal Acid Load Increases Fractional Calcium Absorption and Urinary Calcium Excretion without Affecting Markers of Bone Resorption or Formation in Postmenopausal Women." Journal of Nutrition 141, no. 3 (January 19, 2011): 391-97. http://jn.nutrition.org/content/141/3/391.long.

69. Schwalfenberg, Gerry K. "The Alkaline Diet: Is There Evidence That an Alkaline PH Diet Benefits Health?" Journal of Environmental and Public Health 2012 (October 12, 2011): 1-7. http://www.ncbi.nlm.nih.gov/pmc/articles/PMC3195546/.

70. Deriemaeker, Peter, Dirk Aerenhouts, Marcel Hebbelinck, and Peter Clarys. "Nutrient Based Estimation of Acid-Base Balance in Vegetarians and Non-vegetarians." Plant Foods for Human Nutrition Plant Foods Hum Nutr 65, no. 1 (March 07, 2010): 77-82. http://www.ncbi.nlm.nih.gov/pubmed/20054653.

71. Dawson-Hughes, Bess, Susan S. Harris, and Lisa Ceglia. "Alkaline Diets Favor Lean Tissue Mass in Older Adults." The American Journal of Clinical Nutrition. March 2008. http://www.ncbi.nlm.nih.gov/pmc/articles/PMC2597402/.

72. Chan, June M., Meir J. Stampfer, Jing Ma, Peter H. Gann, J. Michael Gaziano, and Edward L. Giovannucci. "The American Journal of Clinical Nutrition." Dairy Products, Calcium, and Prostate Cancer Risk in the Physicians' Health Study. October 2001. http://ajcn.nutrition.org/content/74/4/549.long.

73. Lanou, A. J. "Should Dairy Be Recommended as Part of a Healthy Vegetarian Diet? Counterpoint." American Journal of Clinical Nutrition 89, no. 5 (March 25, 2009). http://ajcn.nutrition.org/content/89/5/1638S.full.

74. "Milk Consumption and Prostate Cancer." The Physicians Committee. 2010. http://www.pcrm.org/health/health-topics/milk-consumption-and-prostate-cancer.

75. Aune, D., D. A. Navarro Rosenblatt, D. S. Chan, A. R. Vieira, R. Vieira, D. C. Greenwood, L. J. Vatten, and T. Norat. "Dairy Products, Calcium, and Prostate Cancer Risk: A Systematic Review and Meta-analysis of Cohort Studies." American Journal of Clinical Nutrition 101, no. 1 (November 19, 2014): 87-117. http://ajcn.nutrition.org/content/101/1/87.long.

76. Larsson, Susanna C., Nicola Orsini, and Alicja Wolk. "Milk, Milk Products and Lactose Intake and Ovarian Cancer Risk: A Meta-analysis of Epidemiological Studies." International Journal of Cancer Int. J. Cancer 118, no. 2 (July 28, 2005): 431-41. http://onlinelibrary.wiley.com/doi/10.1002/ijc.21305/full.

77. Qin, L-Q, J-Y Xu, P-Y Wang, A. Hashi, K. Hoshi, and A. Sato. "Milk/dairy Products Consumption, Galactose Metabolism and Ovarian Cancer: Meta-analysis of Epidemiological Studies." European Journal of Cancer Prevention 14, no. 1 (February 14, 2005): 13-19. http://www.ncbi.nlm.nih.gov/pubmed/15677891.

78. Keszei, A. P., L. J. Schouten, R. A. Goldbohm, and P. A. Van Den Brandt. "Dairy Intake and the Risk of Bladder Cancer in the Netherlands Cohort Study on Diet and Cancer." American Journal of Epidemiology 171, no. 4 (December 30, 2009): 436-46. http://aje.oxfordjournals.org/content/171/4/436.long.

79. Ganmaa, Davaasambuu, Xiaohui Cui, Diane Feskanich, Susan E. Hankinson, and Walter C. Willett. "Milk, Dairy Intake and Risk of Endometrial Cancer: A 26-year Follow-up." International Journal of Cancer Int. J. Cancer 130, no. 11 (September 17, 2011): 2664-671. http://www.ncbi.nlm.nih.gov/pubmed/21717454.

80. Song, Y., J. E. Chavarro, Y. Cao, W. Qiu, L. Mucci, H. D. Sesso, M. J. Stampfer, E. Giovannucci, M. Pollak, S. Liu, and J. Ma. "Whole Milk Intake Is Associated with Prostate Cancer-Specific Mortality among U.S. Male Physicians." Journal of Nutrition 143, no. 2 (December 19, 2012): 189-96. http://www.ncbi.nlm.nih.gov/pmc/articles/PMC3542910/.

81. Kroenke, C. H., M. L. Kwan, C. Sweeney, A. Castillo, and B. J. Caan. "High- and Low-Fat Dairy Intake, Recurrence, and Mortality After Breast Cancer Diagnosis." JNCI Journal of the National Cancer Institute 105, no. 9 (March 14, 2013): 616-23. http://jnci.oxfordjournals.org/content/early/2013/03/08/jnci.djt027.full.

82. Ganmaa, Davaasambuu, Xiang-Ming Li, Jing Wang, Li-Qiang Qin, Pei-Yu Wang, and Akio Sato. "Incidence and Mortality of Testicular and Prostatic Cancers in Relation to World Dietary Practices." International Journal of Cancer Int. J. Cancer 98, no. 2 (March 10, 2002): 262-67. http://onlinelibrary.wiley.com/doi/10.1002/ijc.10185/full.

83. Garner, Michael J., Nicholas J. Birkett, Kenneth C. Johnson, Bryna Shatenstein, Parviz Ghadirian, and Daniel Krewski. "Dietary Risk Factors for Testicular Carcinoma." International Journal of Cancer Int. J. Cancer 106, no. 6 (June 26, 2003): 934-41. http://onlinelibrary.wiley.com/doi/10.1002/ijc.11327/full.

84. Davies, Tw, Cr Palmer, E. Ruja, and Jm Lipscombe. "Adolescent Milk, Dairy Product and Fruit Consumption and Testicular Cancer." Br J Cancer British Journal of Cancer 74, no. 4 (1996): 657-60. http://www.ncbi.nlm.nih.gov/pmc/articles/PMC2074682/pdf/brjcancer00020-0167.pdf.

85. Pols, J. C Van Der, D. Gunnell, G. M. Williams, J. M P Holly, C. Bain, and R. M. Martin. "Childhood Dairy and Calcium Intake and Cardiovascular Mortality in Adulthood: 65-year Follow-up of the Boyd Orr Cohort." Heart 95, no. 19 (December 2007): 1600-606. http://ajcn.nutrition.org/content/86/6/1722.long.

86. Stang, A., W. Ahrens, C. Baumgardt-Elms, C. Stegmaier, H. Merzenich, M. De Vrese, J. Schrezenmeir, and K.-H. Jockel. "Adolescent Milk Fat and Galactose Consumption and Testicular Germ Cell Cancer." Cancer Epidemiology Biomarkers & Prevention 15, no. 11 (November 15, 2006): 2189-195. http://cebp.aacrjournals.org/content/15/11/2189.full.

87. "Breastfeeding: Human Milk Versus Animal Milk." NutritionMD.org. Accessed February 29, 2016. http://www.nutritionmd.org/nutrition_tips/nutrition_tips_infant_nutrition/breastfeeding_milks.html.

88. Ireland, Corydon. "Hormones in Milk Can Be Dangerous." Hormones in Milk Can Be Dangerous. December 7, 2006. http://news.harvard.edu/gazette/2006/12.07/11-dairy.html.

89. Michaelsson, K., A. Wolk, S. Langenskiold, S. Basu, E. Warensjo Lemming, H. Melhus, and L. Byberg. "Milk Intake and Risk of Mortality and Fractures in Women and Men: Cohort Studies." Bmj 349, no. Oct27 1 (October 28, 2014). http://www.bmj.com/content/349/bmj.g6015.

90. Dizdaroglu, Miral, and Pawel Jaruga. "Mechanisms of Free Radical-induced Damage to DNA." Free Radical Research 46, no. 4 (April 2012): 382-419. http://www.ncbi.nlm.nih.gov/pubmed/22276778.

91. Chen, Xueping, Chunyan Guo, and Jiming Kong. "Oxidative Stress in Neurodegenerative Diseases." Neural Regeneration Research, February 15, 2012, 75-109. http://www.ncbi.nlm.nih.gov/pmc/articles/PMC4350122/.

92. Cui, Xu, Pingping Zuo, Qing Zhang, Xuekun Li, Yazhuo Hu, Jiangang Long, Lester Packer, and Jiankang Liu. "Chronic Systemic D-galactose Exposure Induces Memory Loss, Neurodegeneration, and Oxidative Damage in Mice: Protective Effects of R-⊠-lipoic Acid." J. Neurosci. Res. Journal of Neuroscience Research 83, no. 8 (2006): 1584-590. http://www.student.oulu.fi/~taneliha/Senescence/Chronic systemic D-galactose exposure induces memory loss, neurodegeneration, and oxidative damage in mice, protective effects of R-alpha-lipoic acid.pdf.

93. Larsson, Susanna C., Leif Bergkvist, and Alicja Wolk. "Milk and Lactose Intakes and Ovarian Cancer Risk in the Swedish Mammography Cohort." The American Journal of Clinical Nutrition. November 2004. Accessed March 01, 2016. http://ajcn.nutrition.org/content/80/5/1353.full.

94. "All about the Dairy Group." Choose MyPlate. February 3, 2016. http://www.choosemyplate.gov/dairy.

95. Liebman, Bonnie. "The Changing American Diet: A Report Card." Center for Science in the Public Interest. September 2013. http://cspinet.org/new/pdf/changing_american_diet_13.pdf.

96. Melnik, Bodo C. "Milk: An Epigenetic Amplifier of FTO-mediated Transcription? Implications for Western Diseases." Journal of Translational Medicine J Transl Med 13, no. 1 (December 21, 2015). http://www.ncbi.nlm.nih.gov/pmc/articles/PMC4687119/.

97. Melnik, Bodo. "Milk—A Nutrient System of Mammalian Evolution Promoting MTORC1-Dependent Translation." IJMS International Journal of Molecular Sciences 16, no. 8 (July 27, 2015): 17048-7087. http://www.ncbi.nlm.nih.gov/pmc/articles/PMC4581184/.

98. Melnik, Bodo C., Swen John, and Gerd Schmitz. "Milk Consumption during Pregnancy Increases Birth Weight, a Risk Factor for the Development of Diseases of Civilization." Journal of Translational

Medicine J Transl Med 13, no. 1 (January 16, 2015): 13. http://www.ncbi.nlm.nih.gov/pmc/articles/PMC4302093/.

99. Melnik, Bodo. "The Pathogenic Role of Persistent Milk Signaling in MTORC1- andMilk- MicroRNA-Driven Type 2 Diabetes Mellitus." Current Diabetes Reviews CDR 11, no. 1 (2015): 46-62. http://www.ncbi.nlm.nih.gov/pubmed/25587719.

100. Cromie, William. "Growth Factor Raises Cancer Risk." Growth Factor Raises Cancer Risk. April 29, 1999. http://news.harvard.edu/gazette/1999/04.22/igf1.story.html.

101. Kaaks, Rudolf. "Nutrition, Insulin, IGF-1 Metabolism and Cancer Risk: A Summary of Epidemiological Evidence." Biology of IGF-1: Its Interaction with Insulin in Health and Malignant States Novartis Foundation Symposia, 2004, 247-64. http://www.ncbi.nlm.nih.gov/pubmed/15562834.

102. Giovannucci, Edward. "Insulin, Insulin-Like Growth Factors and Colon Cancer: A Review of the Evidence1." The Journal of Nutrition. November 2001. http://jn.nutrition.org/content/131/11/3109S.long.

103. Furstenberger, G., and H. J. Senn. "Insulin-like Growth Factors and Cancer." May 3, 2002. http://www.ncbi.nlm.nih.gov/pubmed/12067807.

104. Bidosee, M., R. Karry, E. Weiss-Messer, and R. J. Barkey. "Growth Hormone Affects Gene Expression and Proliferation in Human Prostate Cancer Cells." International Journal of Andrology 34, no. 2 (April 2010): 124-37. http://www.ncbi.nlm.nih.gov/pubmed/20546049.

105. Kaaks, Rudolf. "Nutrition, Insulin, IGF-1 Metabolism and Cancer Risk: A Summary of Epidemiological Evidence." Biology of IGF-1: Its Interaction with Insulin in Health and Malignant States Novartis Foundation Symposia, 2004, 247-64. http://www.ncbi.nlm.nih.gov/pubmed/15562834.

106. Clemmons, David R. "Targeting the Insulin-Like Growth Factor-I Receptor in Cancer Therapy." Insulin-like Growth Factors and Cancer, August 10, 2011, 193-213. http://link.springer.com/chapter/10.1007/978-1-4614-0598-6_10.

107. Chan, J. M. "Plasma Insulin-Like Growth Factor-I and Prostate Cancer Risk: A Prospective Study." Science 279, no. 5350 (January 23, 1998): 563-66. http://www.ejnet.org/bgh/igf-1science.html.

108. Hankinson, Susan E., Walter C. Willett, Graham A. Colditz, David J. Hunter, Dominique S. Michaud, Bonnie Deroo, Bernard Rosner, Frank E. Speizer, and Michael Pollak. "Circulating Concentrations of Insulin-like Growth Factor I and Risk of Breast Cancer." The Lancet 351, no. 9113 (May 9, 1998): 1393-396. http://www.sciencedirect.com/science/article/pii/S0140673697103841.

109. Holmes, Michelle D., Michael N. Pollak, Walter C. Willett, and Susan E. Hankinson. "Dietary Correlates of Plasma Insulin-like Growth Factor I and Insulin-like Growth Factor Binding Protein 3 Concentrations1." Cancer Epidemiology, Biomarkers & Prevention. September 11, 2002. http://cebp.aacrjournals.org/content/11/9/852.long.

110. "RBGH: What the Research Shows." Food and Water Watch. August 2007. http://www.foodandwaterwatch.org/sites/default/files/rbgh_what_research_shows_fs_aug_2007.pdf.

111. North, Rick. "FACT SHEET Recombinant Bovine Growth Hormone (rBGH or RBST) Its Documented Harm to Cows." Oregon Physi Cians for Social Responsibility. November 2010. https://www.organicconsumers.org/sites/default/files/rbgh_harms_cows_fact_sheet.pdf.

112. Park, Sung-Woo, Joo-Young Kim, You-Sun Kim, Sang Jin Lee, Sang Don Lee, and Moon Kee Chung. "A Milk Protein, Casein, as a Proliferation Promoting Factor in Prostate Cancer Cells." World J Mens Health The World Journal of Men's Health 32, no. 2 (August 26, 2014): 76. http://www.ncbi.nlm.nih.gov/pmc/articles/PMC4166373/.

113. "Depression." World Health Organization. October 2015. http://www.who.int/mediacentre/factsheets/fs369/en/.

114. Whitaker, Robert. "Now Antidepressant-Induced Chronic Depression Has a Name: Tardive Dysphoria." Psychology Today. June 30, 2011. https://www.psychologytoday.com/blog/mad-in-america/201106/now-antidepressant-induced-chronic-depression-has-name-tardive-dysphoria.

115. Hashmi, Ali Madeeh, Zeeshan Butt, and Muhammad Umair. "Is Depression an Inflammatory Condition? A Review of Available Evidence." Journal of Pakistan Medical Association. July 2013. http://jpma.org.pk/full_article_text.php?article_id=4302.

116. Rosenblat, Joshua D., Danielle S. Cha, Rodrigo B. Mansur, and Roger S. Mcintyre. "Inflamed Moods: A Review of the Interactions

between Inflammation and Mood Disorders." Progress in Neuro-Psychopharmacology and Biological Psychiatry 53 (January 25, 2014): 23-34. http://www.ncbi.nlm.nih.gov/pubmed/24468642.

117. Rosenblat, Joshua D., Elisa Brietzke, Rodrigo B. Mansur, Nadia A. Maruschak, Yena Lee, and Roger S. Mcintyre. "Inflammation as a Neurobiological Substrate of Cognitive Impairment in Bipolar Disorder: Evidence, Pathophysiology and Treatment Implications." Journal of Affective Disorders 188 (December 1, 2015): 149-59. http://www.jad-journal.com/article/S0165-0327(15)30449-3/abstract.

118. Bauer, I. E., M. C. Pascoe, B. Wollenhaupt-Aguiar, F. Kapczinski, and J. C. Soares. "Result Filters." National Center for Biotechnology Information. May 2, 2014. http://www.ncbi.nlm.nih.gov/pubmed/24862657.

119. Benros, Michael E., Berit L. Waltoft, Merete Nordentoft, Søren D. Østergaard, William W. Eaton, Jesper Krogh, and Preben B. Mortensen. "Autoimmune Diseases and Severe Infections as Risk Factors for Mood Disorders." JAMA Psychiatry 70, no. 8 (August 2013): 812. http://archpsyc.jamanetwork.com/article.aspx?articleid=1696348.

120. Eisenberger, Naomi I., Tristen K. Inagaki, Nehjla M. Mashal, and Michael R. Irwin. "Inflammation and Social Experience: An Inflammatory Challenge Induces Feelings of Social Disconnection in Addition to Depressed Mood." Brain, Behavior, and Immunity 24, no. 4 (May 24, 2010): 558-63. http://www.ncbi.nlm.nih.gov/pmc/articles/PMC2856755/.

121. Eisenberger, Naomi I., Elliot T. Berkman, Tristen K. Inagaki, Lian T. Rameson, Nehjla M. Mashal, and Michael R. Irwin. "Inflammation-Induced Anhedonia: Endotoxin Reduces Ventral Striatum Responses to Reward." Biological Psychiatry 68, no. 8 (October 15, 2010): 748-54. http://www.ncbi.nlm.nih.gov/pmc/articles/PMC3025604/.

122. Dellagioia, Nicole, and Jonas Hannestad. "A Critical Review of Human Endotoxin Administration as an Experimental Paradigm of Depression." Neuroscience & Biobehavioral Reviews 34, no. 1 (January 2010): 130-43. http://www.ncbi.nlm.nih.gov/pmc/articles/PMC2795398/.

123. Lucas, Michel, Patricia Chocano-Bedoya, Mathias B. Shulze, Fariba Mirzaei, Éilis J. O'Reilly, Olivia I. Okereke, Frank B. Hu, Walter C. Willett, and Alberto Ascherio. "Inflammatory Dietary Pattern and Risk

of Depression among Women." Brain, Behavior, and Immunity 36 (February 2014): 46-53. http://www.ncbi.nlm.nih.gov/pmc/articles/PMC3947176/.

124. Garcia-Calzon, S., G. Zalba, M. Ruiz-Canela, N. Shivappa, J. R. Hebert, J. A. Martinez, M. Fito, E. Gomez-Gracia, M. A. Martinez-Gonzalez, and A. Marti. "Dietary Inflammatory Index and Telomere Length in Subjects with a High Cardiovascular Disease Risk from the PREDIMED-NAVARRA Study: Cross-sectional and Longitudinal Analyses over 5 Y." American Journal of Clinical Nutrition 102, no. 4 (September 09, 2015): 897-904. http://www.pubfacts.com/detail/26354530/Dietary-inflammatory-index-and-telomere-length-in-subjects-with-a-high-cardiovascular-disease-risk-f.

125. Muller, Norbert. "The Role Of Anti-inflammatory Treatment In Psychiatric Disorders." Department of Psychiatry and Psychotherapy, Ludwig-Maximilian University Munich, Munich, Germany. 2013. http://www.hdbp.org/psychiatria_danubina/pdf/dnb_vol25_no3/dnb_vol25_no3_292.pdf.

126. Agarwal, Ulka, MD. "Foods That Fight Depression." The Physicians Committee. February 27, 2015. http://www.pcrm.org/nbBlog/index.php/foods-that-fight-depression.

127. Hoppner, Karl. "I Went Plant-Based and Left Life-Threatening Depression Behind." Forks Over Knives. January 18, 2016. http://www.forksoverknives.com/i-went-plant-based-and-left-life-threatening-depression-behind/?mc_cid=ab4c02ced0.

128. Greger, Michael, MD. "NutritionFacts.org." NutritionFactsorg. Accessed March 02, 2016. http://nutritionfacts.org/?s=depression.

129. Brandel, Jean-Philippe, Craig A. Heath, Mark W. Head, Etienne Levavasseur, Richard Knight, Jean-Louis Laplanche, Jan Pm. Langeveld, James W. Ironside, Jean-Jacques Hauw, Jan Mackenzie, Annick Alpérovitch, Robert G. Will, and Stéphane Haïk. "Variant Creutzfeldt-Jakob Disease in France and the United Kingdom: Evidence for the Same Agent Strain." Annals of Neurology Ann Neurol. 65, no. 3 (March 2009): 249-56. http://www.ncbi.nlm.nih.gov/pubmed/19334063.

130. Diack, Abigail B., Mark W. Head, Sandra Mccutcheon, Aileen Boyle, Richard Knight, James W. Ironside, Jean C. Manson, and Robert G. Will. "Variant CJD." Prion 8, no. 4 (2014): 286-95. http://www.ncbi.nlm.nih.

gov/pubmed/25495404.

131. Prusiner, S. B. "Prion Diseases and the BSE Crisis." Science 278, no.
5336 (1997): 245-51. http://www.sciencemag.org/site/feature/data/
prusiner/245.xhtml.

132. "Center for Food Safety | News Room | California Cows Unhappy About
Mad Cow Disease." Center for Food Safety. April 25, 2012. http://www.
centerforfoodsafety.org/press-releases/706/california-cows-unhappy-about-
mad-cow-disease.

133. Lupkin, Sydney. "4 Things to Know About Mad Cow Disease." ABC
News. June 6, 2014. http://abcnews.go.com/Health/things-mad-cow-
disease/story?id=24027370.

134. "Confirmed Variant Creutzfeldt-Jakob Disease (variant CJD) Case in
Texas." Centers for Disease Control and Prevention. October 7, 2014.
http://www.cdc.gov/ncidod/dvrd/vcjd/other/confirmed-case-in-texas.htm.

135. Ramel, A., J. A. Martinez, M. Kiely, N. M. Bandarra, and I. Thorsdottir.
"Effects of Weight Loss and Seafood Consumption on Inflammation
Parameters in Young, Overweight and Obese European Men and Women
during 8 Weeks of Energy Restriction." European Journal of Clinical
Nutrition Eur J Clin Nutr 64, no. 9 (June 16, 2010): 987-93. http://www.
ncbi.nlm.nih.gov/pubmed/20551965.

136. Ramel, A., J. A. Martinez, M. Kiely, N. M. Bandarra, and I. Thorsdottir.
"Effects of Weight Loss and Seafood Consumption on Inflammation
Parameters in Young, Overweight and Obese European Men and Women
during 8 Weeks of Energy Restriction." European Journal of Clinical
Nutrition Eur J Clin Nutr 64, no. 9 (June 16, 2010): 987-93. http://www.
ncbi.nlm.nih.gov/pubmed/20551965.

137. Kaushik, M., D. Mozaffarian, D. Spiegelman, J. E. Manson, W. C.
Willett, and F. B. Hu. "Long-chain Omega-3 Fatty Acids, Fish Intake,
and the Risk of Type 2 Diabetes Mellitus." American Journal of Clinical
Nutrition 90, no. 3 (July 22, 2009): 613-20. http://www.ncbi.nlm.nih.
gov/pubmed/19625683.

138. "American Seafood: Something's Fishy." The Physicians Committee. 2014.
http://www.pcrm.org/health/reports/american-seafood-somethings-fishy.

139. Karimi, Roxanne, Caterina Vacchi-Suzzi, and Jaymie R. Meliker.
"Mercury Exposure and a Shift toward Oxidative Stress in Avid Seafood

Consumers." Environmental Research 146 (December 30, 2015): 100-07. http://www.ncbi.nlm.nih.gov/pubmed/26745733.

140. Norat, T., S. Bingham, and E. Riboli. "RESPONSE: Re: Meat, Fish, and Colorectal Cancer Risk: The European Prospective Investigation into Cancer and Nutrition." JNCI Journal of the National Cancer Institute 97, no. 23 (June 15, 2005): 1788-789. http://www.ncbi.nlm.nih.gov/pubmed/15956652.

141. Stripp, C., K. Overvad, J. Christensen, B. L. Thomsen, A. Olsen, S. Moller, and A. Tjonneland. "Result Filters." National Center for Biotechnology Information. November 2003. http://www.ncbi.nlm.nih.gov/pubmed/14608091.

142. Malter, Jordan, Robert Sevilla, and Kate Trafecante. "How the Animals You Eat Get Fat." CNNMoney. Cable News Network. Web. <http://money.cnn.com/video/news/economy/2016/01/10/raw-ingredients-how-the-animals-you-eat-get-fat.cnnmoney/>.

143. "Import Alert 16-131." U.S. Food and Drug Administration. February 29, 2016. http://www.accessdata.fda.gov/cms_ia/importalert_33.html.

144. "Requirements for Importation of Fish and Fish Product under the U.S. Marine Mammal Protection Act." Federal Register. 2014. https://www.federalregister.gov/regulations/0648-AY15/requirements-for-importation-of-fish-and-fish-product-under-the-u-s-marine-mammal-protection-act.

145. "Living Blue Planet Report: Species, Habitats and Human Well-being." World Wildlife Fund. 2015. http://assets.worldwildlife.org/publications/817/files/original/Living_Blue_Planet_Report_2015_Final_LR.pdf?1442242821&_ga=1.215677015.1317319810.1457034412.

146. "PCBs in Farmed Salmon." Environmental Working Group. July 31, 2003. http://www.ewg.org/research/pcbs-farmed-salmon.

147. "Health Effects of PCBs." Environmental Protection Agency. February 22, 2016. http://www3.epa.gov/epawaste/hazard/tsd/pcbs/pubs/effects.htm.

148. "OEHHA Fish: PCBs." Ca.gov Office of Environmental Health Hazard Assessment. Accessed March 03, 2016. http://oehha.ca.gov/fish/pcb/.

149. "The Catch With Seafood: Human Health Impacts of Drugs and

Chemicals Used by the Aquaculture Industry." Center for Food Safety. 2005. http://www.centerforfoodsafety.org/files/aquaculture-reportfinal672005_35761.pdf.

150. Evensen, Øystein, and Jo-Ann C. Leong. "DNA Vaccines against Viral Diseases of Farmed Fish." Fish & Shellfish Immunology 35, no. 6 (October 31, 2013): 1751-758. http://www.ncbi.nlm.nih.gov/pubmed/24184267.

151. Crane, Mark, and Alex Hyatt. "Viruses of Fish: An Overview of Significant Pathogens." Viruses 3, no. 12 (October 25, 2011): 2025-046. http://www.ncbi.nlm.nih.gov/pubmed/22163333. \

152. "Human Vaccines to Aid Farmed Fish." Sciencenordic.com. September 9, 2014. http://sciencenordic.com/human-vaccines-aid-farmed-fish.

Planet Earth

1. "Fifth Assessment Report - Mitigation of Climate Change." Intergovernmental Panel on Climate Change. 2014. http://www.ipcc.ch/report/ar5/wg3/.

2. "A More Potent Greenhouse Gas than Carbon Dioxide, Methane Emissions Will Leap as Earth Warms." ScienceDaily. March 27, 2014. https://www.sciencedaily.com/releases/2014/03/140327111724.htm.

3. "World Population Prospects." United Nations. 2015. http://esa.un.org/unpd/wpp/Publications/Files/Key_Findings_WPP_2015.pdf.

4. Palmer, Brian. "Our Oceans Are Full of Dead Zones. Climate Change Makes Them...deader." OnEarth. 2014. http://www.onearth.org/earthwire/devil-deep-blue-sea.

5. "Factory Farms." Environmental Integrity Project. Accessed March 04, 2016. http://environmentalintegrity.org/issue-areas/factory-farms.

6. "Facts about Pollution from Livestock Farms." Natural Resources Defense Council. February 21, 2013. http://www.nrdc.org/water/pollution/ffarms.asp.

7. "Coalition Sues EPA for Failing to Address Factory Farm Air Pollution." Environmental Integrity Project. January 28, 2015. http://environmentalintegrity.org/archives/7147.

8. "Pig Factory Sued for Keeping Community in Dark About Hazardous Pollutants." The Humane Society of the United States. July 1, 2015. http://www.humanesociety.org/news/press_releases/2015/07/factory-farm-sued-ammonia-070115.html.

9. Hamilton, T. D. C., J. M. Roe, C. M. Hayes, and A. J. F. Webster. "Effects of Ammonia Inhalation and Acetic Acid Pretreatment on Colonization Kinetics of Toxigenic Pasteurella Multocida within Upper Respiratory Tracts of Swine." Journal of Clinical Microbiology. May 1998. http://www.ncbi.nlm.nih.gov/pmc/articles/PMC104811/.

10. "Livestock a Major Threat to Environment." Food and Agriculture Organization of the United Nations. November 29, 2006. http://www.fao.org/newsroom/en/News/2006/1000448/index.html.

11. "Production and Trade of All Meats to Expand in 2016." United States Department of Agriculture. October 2015. http://apps.fas.usda.gov/psdonline/circulars/livestock_poultry.PDF.

12. "Restoration and Spending Plan Marks Farm Natural Resource Damages Settlement." New York State Department of Environmental Conservation. November 7, 2014. http://www.dec.ny.gov/docs/fish_marine_pdf/mfarmresplfin.pdf.

13. Bauer, Angela C., Sarah Wingert, Kevin J. Fermanich, and Michael E. Zorn. "Well Water in Karst Regions of Northeastern Wisconsin Contains Estrogenic Factors, Nitrate, and Bacteria." Water Environment Research 85, no. 4 (April 2013): 318-26. http://www.ncbi.nlm.nih.gov/pubmed/23697235.

14. "Wisconsin Groups Demand Investigation of Drinking Water Contamination from Factory Dairy." Environmental Integrity Project. April 8, 2015. http://environmentalintegrity.org/archives/7227.

15. Onsrud, Aaron, Et Al. "Missouri River Basin (Upper Big Sioux, Lower Big Sioux, Little Sioux, and Rock River Watersheds) Monitoring and Assessment Report." Minnesota Pollution Control Agency. September 2014. https://www.pca.state.mn.us/sites/default/files/wq-ws3-10170204b.pdf.

16. "Facts and Sources." COWSPIRACY. 2014. http://www.cowspiracy.com/facts/.

17. Rudolf, John Collins. "Murder of Activists Raises Questions of Justice

in Amazon." Green Blog. May 28, 2011. http://green.blogs.nytimes. com/2011/05/28/murder-of-amazon-activists-raises-justice-questions/?rref=collection/timestopic/Stang, Sister Dorothy.

A Modern Myth

1. "The Protein Myth." The Physicians Committee. Accessed March 04, 2016. http://www.pcrm.org/health/diets/vsk/vegetarian-starter-kit-protein.

2. Novick, Jeff, MS,RD. "The Myth of Complementary Protein." Forks Over Knives. June 03, 2013. http://www.forksoverknives.com/the-myth-of-complementary-protein/.

3. Nestle, Marion. Food Politics: How the Food Industry Influences Nutrition and
    Health. Berkeley, CA: University of California Press, 2013.

4. "National Dairy Council." SourceWatch. January 17, 2011. http:// www.sourcewatch.org/index.php/National_Dairy_Council.

5. "USDA Mission Areas | USDA." United States Department of Agriculture. Accessed March 04, 2016. http://www.usda.gov/wps/ portal/usda/usdahome?navid=USDA_MISSION_AREAS.

6. "USDA Dietary Guidelines." SourceWatch. July 15, 2011. http:// www.sourcewatch.org/index.php/USDA_Dietary_Guidelines.

7. "The Physicians Committee Sues USDA and DHHS, Exposing Industry Corruption in Dietary Guidelines Decision on Cholesterol." The Physicians Committee. January 06, 2016. https://www.pcrm.org/ media/news/physicians-committee-sues-usda-and-dhhs.

8. Popkin, Barry M., Linda S. Adair, and Shu Wen Ng. "Global Nutrition Transition and the Pandemic of Obesity in Developing Countries." Nutrition Reviews 70, no. 1 (January 2012): 3-21. http:// www.ncbi.nlm.nih.gov/pmc/articles/PMC3257829/.

9. Elsevier. "Following a Western style diet may lead to greater risk of premature death." ScienceDaily. www.sciencedaily.com/ releases/2013/04/130415124542.htm (accessed March 4, 2016).

10. Ward, Wendy E., Susie Kim, and W. Robert Bruce. "A Western-style Diet Reduces Bone Mass and Biomechanical Bone

Strength to a Greater Extent in Male Compared with Female Rats during Development." *BJN British Journal of Nutrition 90*, no. 03 (September 2003): 589. http://www.ncbi.nlm.nih.gov/ pubmed/13129465.

11. Odegaard, A. O., W. P. Koh, J.-M. Yuan, M. D. Gross, and M. A. Pereira. "Western-Style Fast Food Intake and Cardiometabolic Risk in an Eastern Country." Circulation 126, no. 2 (July 02, 2012): 182-88. http://circ.ahajournals.org/content/126/2/182.full.

12. Buettner, Dan. *The Blue Zones: Lessons for Living Longer from the People Who've Lived the Longest.* Washington, D.C.: National Geographic Society, 2009.

Family Affair

1. Anand, Preetha, Ajaikumar B. Kunnumakkara, Chitra Sundaram, Kuzhuvelil B. Harikumar, Sheeja T. Tharakan, Oiki S. Lai, Bokyung Sung, and Bharat B. Aggarwal. "Cancer Is a Preventable Disease That Requires Major Lifestyle Changes." Pharm Res Pharmaceutical Research 25, no. 9 (July 15, 2008): 2200. http://www.ncbi.nlm.nih. gov/pmc/articles/PMC2515569/.

2. Ford, E. S., M. M. Bergmann, J. Kroger, A. Schienkiewitz, C. Weikert, and H. Boeing. "Healthy Living Is the Best Revenge." Arch Intern Med Archives of Internal Medicine 169, no. 15 (August 10, 2009): 1355. http://www.ncbi.nlm.nih.gov/pubmed/19667296/.

3. Gonzalez, Carlos A., and Elio Riboli. "Diet and Cancer Prevention: Contributions from the European Prospective Investigation into Cancer and Nutrition (EPIC) Study." European Journal of Cancer 46, no. 14 (September 2010): 2555-562. http://www.ncbi.nlm.nih. gov/pubmed/20843485.

4. Bamia, C., P. Lagiou, M. Jenab, K. Aleksandrova, V. Fedirko, D. Trichopoulos, K. Overvad, A. Tjønneland, A. Olsen, F. Clavel-Chapelon, M-C Boutron-Ruault, M. Kvaskoff, V. A. Katzke, T. Kühn, H. Boeing, U. Nöthlings, D. Palli, S. Sieri, S. Panico, R. Tumino, A. Naccarati, Hb(As) Bueno-De-Mesquita, P. H M Peeters, E. Weiderpass, G. Skeie, J. R. Quirós, A. Agudo, M-D Chirlaque, M-J Sanchez, E. Ardanaz, M. Dorronsoro, U. Ericson, L. M. Nilsson, M. Wennberg, K-T Khaw, N. Wareham, T. J. Key, R. C. Travis,

REFERENCES

P. Ferrari, M. Stepien, T. Duarte-Salles, T. Norat, N. Murphy, E. Riboli, and A. Trichopoulou. "Fruit and Vegetable Consumption in Relation to Hepatocellular Carcinoma in a Multi-centre, European Cohort Study." Br J *Cancer British Journal of Cancer* 112, no. 7 (March 31, 2015): 1273-282. http://www.ncbi.nlm.nih.gov/pubmed/25742480?&report=abstract.

5. Murray, J.a. "Diet and Risk of Diverticular Disease in Oxford Cohort of European Prospective Investigation into Cancer and Nutrition (EPIC): Prospective Study of British Vegetarians and Non-vegetarians." *Yearbook of Medicine* 2012 (July 19, 2011): 407-08. http://www.ncbi.nlm.nih.gov/pubmed/21771850.

6. Park, Jin Young, H.b(As) Bueno-De-Mesquita, Pietro Ferrari, Paolo Vineis, Elisabete Weiderpass, and Nadia Slimani. "Abstract 4811: Dietary Folate Intake and Pancreatic Cancer Risk: Results from the European Prospective Investigation into Cancer and Nutrition." *Cancer Research Cancer Res* 73, no. 8 Supplement (November 12, 2014): 4811. http://www.ncbi.nlm.nih.gov/pubmed/25505228?&report=abstract.

7. Goff, L. M., J. D. Bell, P-W So, A. Dornhorst, and G. S. Frost. "Veganism and Its Relationship with Insulin Resistance and Intramyocellular Lipid." *European Journal of Clinical Nutrition Eur J Clin Nutr* 59, no. 2 (February 2005): 291-98. http://www.ncbi.nlm.nih.gov/pubmed/15523486.

8. Gojda, J., J. Patková, M. Jaček, J. Potočková, J. Trnka, P. Kraml, and M. Aněl. "Higher Insulin Sensitivity in Vegans Is Not Associated with Higher Mitochondrial Density." *European Journal of Clinical Nutrition Eur J Clin Nutr* 67, no. 12 (December 23, 2013): 1310-315. http://www.ncbi.nlm.nih.gov/pubmed/24149445.

9. Sandler, R. S., C. M. Lyles, L. A. Peipins, C. A. Mcauliffe, J. T. Woosley, and L. L. Kupper. "Diet and Risk of Colorectal Adenomas: Macronutrients, Cholesterol, and Fiber." *JNCI Journal of the National Cancer Institute* 85, no. 11 (June 02, 1993): 884-91. http://www.ncbi.nlm.nih.gov/pubmed/8388061.

10. Nagura, Junko, Hiroyasu Iso, Yoshiyuki Watanabe, Koutatsu Maruyama, Chigusa Date, Hideaki Toyoshima, Akio Yamamoto, Shogo Kikuchi, Akio Koizumi, Takaaki Kondo, Yasuhiko Wada,

Yutaka Inaba, and Akiko Tamakoshi. "Fruit, Vegetable and Bean Intake and Mortality from Cardiovascular Disease among Japanese Men and Women: The JACC Study." *BJN British Journal of Nutrition* 102, no. 02 (January 13, 2009):285. http://journals.cambridge.org/action/

11. Eshak, E. S., H. Iso, C. Date, S. Kikuchi, Y. Watanabe, Y. Wada, K. Wakai, and A. Tamakoshi. "Dietary Fiber Intake Is Associated with Reduced Risk of Mortality from Cardiovascular Disease among Japanese Men and Women." *Journal of Nutrition* 140, no. 8 (June 23, 2010): 1445-1453. http://www.ncbi.nlm.nih.gov/pubmed/20573945.

12. Park, S.-Y., N. J. Ollberding, C. G. Woolcott, L. R. Wilkens, B. E. Henderson, and L. N. Kolonel. "Fruit and Vegetable Intakes Are Associated with Lower Risk of Bladder Cancer among Women in the Multiethnic Cohort Study." *Journal of Nutrition* 143, no. 8 (June 05, 2013): 1283-292. http://jn.nutrition.org/content/143/8/1283.abstract.

13. Lian, F., J. Wang, X. Huang, Y. Wu, Y. Cao, X. Tan, X. Xu, Y. Hong, L. Yang, and X. Gao. "Effect of Vegetable Consumption on the Association between Peripheral Leucocyte Telomere Length and Hypertension: A Case-control Study." *BMJ Open* 5, no. 11 (November 11, 2015). http://bmjopen.bmj.com/content/5/11/e009305?cpetoc&trendmd-shared=0.

14. Miedema, Michael D., Andrew Petrone, James Shikany, Philip Greenland, Cora Lewis, Mark Pletcher, J. Michael Gaziano, and Luc Djousse. "The Association Of Fruit And Vegetable Consumption During Early Adulthood With The Prevalence Of Coronary Artery Calcium After 20 Years Of Follow-Up: The Coronary Artery Risk Development In Young Adults (Cardia) Study." *Journal of the American College of Cardiology* 63, no. 12 (November 24, 2014). http://www.ncbi.nlm.nih.gov/pubmed/26503880.

15. Martínez-González, Miguel Á, Carmen De La Fuente-Arrillaga, Cristina López-Del-Burgo, Zenaida Vázquez-Ruiz, Silvia Benito, and Miguel Ruiz-Canela. "Low Consumption of Fruit and Vegetables and Risk of Chronic Disease: A Review of the Epidemiological Evidence and Temporal Trends among Spanish Graduates." *Public Health Nutr. Public Health Nutrition* 14, no. 12A (December 2011): 2309-315. http://www.ncbi.nlm.nih.gov/pubmed/22166189.

16. Chen, Y. M., S. C. Ho, and J. L. Woo. "Result Filters." National Center for Biotechnology Information. October 2006. http://www.ncbi.nlm.nih.gov/pubmed/17010235.

17. Butler, L. M., A. H. Wu, R. Wang, W.-P. Koh, J.-M. Yuan, and M. C. Yu. "A Vegetable-fruit-soy Dietary Pattern Protects against Breast Cancer among Postmenopausal Singapore Chinese Women." *American Journal of Clinical Nutrition* 91, no. 4 (April 2010): 1013-019. http://www.ncbi.nlm.nih.gov/pubmed/20181808.

18. Liu, Zhao-Min, Jason Leung, Samuel Yeung-Shan Wong, Carmen Ka Man Wong, Ruth Chan, and Jean Woo. "Greater Fruit Intake Was Associated With Better Bone Mineral Status Among Chinese Elderly Men and Women: Results of Hong Kong Mr. Os and Ms. Os Studies." Journal of the American Medical Directors Association 16, no. 4 (April 2015): 309-15. http://www.ncbi.nlm.nih.gov/pubmed/25523283.

19. Li, Jing-Jing, Zhen-Wu Huang, Ruo-Qin Wang, Xiao-Ming Ma, Zhe-Qing Zhang, Zen Liu, Yu-Ming Chen, and Yi-Xiang Su. "Fruit and Vegetable Intake and Bone Mass in Chinese Adolescents, Young and Postmenopausal Women." Public Health Nutr. Public Health Nutrition 16, no. 01 (April 17, 2012): 78-86. http://www.ncbi.nlm.nih.gov/pubmed/22717072.

20. Steffen, Lyn M., Candyce H. Kroenke, Xinhua Yu, Mark A. Pereira, Martha L. Slattery, Linda Van Horn, Myron D. Gross, and David R. Jacobs, Jr. "The American Journal of Clinical Nutrition." Associations of Plant Food, Dairy Product, and Meat Intakes with 15-y Incidence of Elevated Blood Pressure in Young Black and White Adults: The Coronary Artery Risk Development in Young Adults (CARDIA) Study. December 2005. http://ajcn.nutrition.org/content/82/6/1169.long.

21. Cassidy, A., M. Franz, and E. B. Rimm. "Dietary Flavonoid Intake and Incidence of Erectile Dysfunction." American Journal of Clinical Nutrition 103, no. 2 (January 13, 2016): 534-41. http://ajcn.nutrition.org/content/early/2016/01/06/ajcn.115.122010.abstract.

22. Rumawas, Marcella E., Nicola M. Mckeown, Gail Rogers, James B. Meigs, Peter W.f. Wilson, and Paul F. Jacques. "Magnesium Intake Is Related to Improved Insulin Homeostasis in the Framingham

Offspring Cohort." Journal of the American College of Nutrition 25, no. 6 (December 2006): 486-92. http://www.ncbi.nlm.nih.gov/pubmed/17229895.

23. Murakami, Kentaro, Hitomi Okubo, and Satoshi Sasaki. "Effect of Dietary Factors on Incidence of Type 2 Diabetes: A Systematic Review of Cohort Studies." Journal of Nutritional Science and Vitaminology, J Nutr Sci Vitaminol Journal of Nutritional Science and Vitaminology 51, no. 4 (August 2005): 292-310. http://www.ncbi.nlm.nih.gov/pubmed/16262005.

24. Wang, Jinsong, Gioia Persuitte, Barbara Olendzki, Nicole Wedick, Zhiying Zhang, Philip Merriam, Hua Fang, James Carmody, Gin-Fei Olendzki, and Yunsheng Ma. "Dietary Magnesium Intake Improves Insulin Resistance among Non-Diabetic Individuals with Metabolic Syndrome Participating in a Dietary Trial." Nutrients 5, no. 10 (September 27, 2013): 3910-919. http://www.mdpi.com/2072-6643/5/10/3910.

25. London, Mark. "The Role of Magnesium in Fibromyalgia." Massachusettes Institute of Technology. 2007. http://web.mit.edu/london/www/magnesium.html.

26. Le, Lap, and Joan Sabaté. "Beyond Meatless, the Health Effects of Vegan Diets: Findings from the Adventist Cohorts." Nutrients 6, no. 6 (May 27, 2014): 2131-147. http://www.ncbi.nlm.nih.gov/pmc/articles/PMC4073139/.

27. Craig, W. J. "Health Effects of Vegan Diets." American Journal of Clinical Nutrition 89, no. 5 (March 11, 2009). http://ajcn.nutrition.org/content/89/5/1627S.full.

28. Tonstad, Serena, Edward Nathan, Keiji Oda, and Gary Fraser. "Vegan Diets and Hypothyroidism." Nutrients 5, no. 11 (November 20, 2013): 4642-652. http://www.ncbi.nlm.nih.gov/pubmed/24264226.

29. Dinu, Monica, Rosanna Abbate, Gian Franco Gensini, Alessandro Casini, and Francesco Sofi. "Vegetarian, Vegan Diets and Multiple Health Outcomes: A Systematic Review with Meta-analysis of Observational Studies." Critical Reviews in Food Science and Nutrition, February 06, 2016, 00. http://www.ncbi.nlm.nih.gov/pubmed/26853923.

30. Barnard, N. D., J. Cohen, D. J. Jenkins, G. Turner-Mcgrievy, L. Gloede, A. /Green, and H. Ferdowsian. "A Low-fat Vegan Diet and a Conventional Diabetes Diet in the Treatment of Type 2 Diabetes: A Randomized, Controlled, 74-wk Clinical Trial." American Journal of Clinical Nutrition 89, no. 5 (April 01, 2009). http://www.ncbi.nlm.nih.gov/pubmed/19339401.

31. Dewell, Antonella, Gerdi Weidner, Michael D. Sumner, Christine S. Chi, and Dean Ornish. "A Very-Low-Fat Vegan Diet Increases Intake of Protective Dietary Factors and Decreases Intake of Pathogenic Dietary Factors." Journal of the American Dietetic Association 108, no. 2 (2008): 347-56. http://www.ornishspectrum.com/wp-content/uploads/A-Very-Low-Fat-Vegan-Diet-Increases.pdf.

32. Afshin, A., R. Micha, S. Khatibzadeh, and D. Mozaffarian. "Consumption of Nuts and Legumes and Risk of Incident Ischemic Heart Disease, Stroke, and Diabetes: A Systematic Review and Meta-analysis." American Journal of Clinical Nutrition 100, no. 1 (June 04, 2014): 278-88. http://ajcn.nutrition.org/content/100/1/278.

33. Kang, Jae H., Walter C. Willett, Bernard A. Rosner, Emmanuel Buys, Janey L. Wiggs, and Louis R. Pasquale. "Association of Dietary Nitrate Intake With Primary Open-Angle Glaucoma." JAMA Ophthalmol JAMA Ophthalmology, January 14, 2016, 1. http://www.ncbi.nlm.nih.gov/pubmed/26767881.

34. Larsson, S. C., L. Holmberg, and A. Wolk. "Fruit and Vegetable Consumption in Relation to Ovarian Cancer Incidence: The Swedish Mammography Cohort." Br J Cancer British Journal of Cancer, June 1, 2004. http://www.ncbi.nlm.nih.gov/pubmed/15150575.

35. Wang, X., Y. Ouyang, J. Liu, M. Zhu, G. Zhao, W. Bao, and F. B. Hu. "Fruit and Vegetable Consumption and Mortality from All Causes, Cardiovascular Disease, and Cancer: Systematic Review and Dose-response Meta-analysis of Prospective Cohort Studies." Bmj 349, no. Sep03 18 (July 29, 2014). http://www.ncbi.nlm.nih.gov/pubmed/25073782.

36. Grosso, G., J. Yang, S. Marventano, A. Micek, F. Galvano, and S. N. Kales. "Nut Consumption on All-cause, Cardiovascular, and Cancer Mortality Risk: A Systematic Review and Meta-analysis of Epidemiologic Studies." American Journal of Clinical Nutrition 101,

no. 4 (February 04, 2015): 783-93. http://www.ncbi.nlm.nih.gov/pubmed/25833976.

37. Cocate, P. G., A. J. Natali, R. C. G. Alfenas, A. De Oliveira, E. C. Dos Santos, and H. H. M. Hermsdorff. "Carotenoid Consumption Is Related to Lower Lipid Oxidation and DNA Damage in Middle-aged Men." British Journal of Nutrition Br J Nutr 114, no. 02 (April 14, 2015): 257-64. http://www.silae.it/files/S0007114515001622a.pdf.

38. Jung, Seungyoun, and Stephanie A. Smith-Warner. "Abstract 3719: Fruit and Vegetable Intake and Risk of Breast Cancer Characterized by Estrogen Receptor (ER) and Progesterone Receptor (PR) Status." Cancer Research Cancer Res 71, no. 8 Supplement (January 24, 2013): 3719. http://jnci.oxfordjournals.org/content/early/2013/01/18/jnci.djs635.full.

39. Bakker, M. F., P. H. Peeters, V. M. Klaasen, H. B. Bueno-De-Mesquita, E. H. Jansen, M. M. Ros, N. Travier, A. Olsen, A. Tjonneland, K. Overvad, S. Rinaldi, I. Romieu, P. Brennan, M.-C. Boutron-Ruault, F. Perquier, C. Cadeau, H. Boeing, K. Aleksandrova, R. Kaaks, T. Ku Hn, A. Trichopoulou, P. Lagiou, D. Trichopoulos, P. Vineis, V. Krogh, S. Panico, G. Masala, R. Tumino, E. Weiderpass, G. Skeie, E. Lund, J. R. Quiros, E. Ardanaz, C. Navarro, P. Amiano, M.-J. Sanchez, G. Buckland, U. Ericson, E. Sonestedt, M. Johansson, M. Sund, R. C. Travis, T. J. Key, K.-T. Khaw, N. Wareham, E. Riboli, and C. H. Van Gils. "Plasma Carotenoids, Vitamin C, Tocopherols, and Retinol and the Risk of Breast Cancer in the European Prospective Investigation into Cancer and Nutrition Cohort,." American Journal of Clinical Nutrition 103, no. 2 (January 20, 2016): 454-64. http://ajcn.nutrition.org/content/103/2/454.abstract?sid=44ad585c-3851-43b7-b9c4-97451ad2c70b.

40. Goldsmith, Jason R., and R. Balfour Sartor. "The Role of Diet on Intestinal Microbiota Metabolism: Downstream Impacts on Host Immune Function and Health, and Therapeutic Implications." Journal of Gastroenterology J Gastroenterol 49, no. 5 (March 21, 2014): 785-98. http://www.ncbi.nlm.nih.gov/pubmed/24652102.

41. Minihane, Anne M., Sophie Vinoy, Wendy R. Russell, Athanasia Baka, Helen M. Roche, Kieran M. Tuohy, Jessica L. Teeling, Ellen E. Blaak, Michael Fenech, David Vauzour, Harry J. Mcardle, Bas

REFERENCES

H. A. Kremer, Luc Sterkman, Katerina Vafeiadou, Massimo Massi Benedetti, Christine M. Williams, and Philip C. Calder. "Low-grade Inflammation, Diet Composition and Health: Current Research Evidence and Its Translation." British Journal of Nutrition Br J Nutr 114, no. 07 (July 31, 2015): 999-1012. http://www.ncbi.nlm.nih.gov/pmc/articles/PMC4579563/.

42. Soory, Mena. "Nutritional Antioxidants and Their Applications in Cardiometabolic Diseases." IDDT Infectious Disorders - Drug Targets 12, no. 5 (October 2012): 388-401. http://www.ncbi.nlm.nih.gov/pubmed/23167714.

43. Soory, Mena. "Relevance of Nutritional Antioxidants in Metabolic Syndrome, Ageing and Cancer: Potential for Therapeutic Targeting." IDDT Infectious Disorders - Drug Targets 9, no. 4 (2009): 400-14. http://www.eurekaselect.com/84685/article?trendmd-shared=0.

44. Daglia, Maria, Arianna Lorenzo, Seyed Nabavi, Zeliha Talas, and Seyed Nabavi. "Polyphenols: Well Beyond The Antioxidant Capacity: Gallic Acid and Related Compounds as Neuroprotective Agents: You Are What You Eat!" Current Pharmaceutical Biotechnology CPB 15, no. 4 (2014): 362-72. http://www.ncbi.nlm.nih.gov/pubmed/24938889.

45. Kelsey, Natalie A., Heather M. Wilkins, and Daniel A. Linseman. "Nutraceutical Antioxidants as Novel Neuroprotective Agents." Molecules 15, no. 11 (November 03, 2010): 7792-814. http://www.ncbi.nlm.nih.gov/pubmed/21060289.

46. Wang, Jia-Yi, Li- Li Wen, Ya-Ni Huang, Yen-Tsun Chen, and Min-Chi Ku. "Dual Effects of Antioxidants in Neurodegeneration: Direct Neuroprotection against Oxidative Stress and Indirect Protection via Suppression of Gliamediated Inflammation." CPD Current Pharmaceutical Design 12, no. 27 (2006): 3521-533. http://www.ncbi.nlm.nih.gov/pubmed/17017945.

47. Poljsak, B., and I. Milisav. "Aging, Oxidative Stress and Antioxidants." Oxidative Stress and Chronic Degenerative Diseases - A Role for Antioxidants, December 1999. http://www.ncbi.nlm.nih.gov/pubmed/10601882.

48. David, Lawrence A., Corinne F. Maurice, Rachel N. Carmody, David B. Gootenberg, Julie E. Button, Benjamin E. Wolfe, Alisha V.

Ling, A. Sloan Devlin, Yug Varma, Michael A. Fischbach, Sudha B. Biddinger, Rachel J. Dutton, and Peter J. Turnbaugh. "Diet Rapidly and Reproducibly Alters the Human Gut Microbiome." Nature 505, no. 7484 (December 11, 2013): 559-63. http://www.ncbi.nlm.nih. gov/pmc/articles/PMC3957428/.

49. Filippo, C. De, D. Cavalieri, M. Di Paola, M. Ramazzotti, J. B. Poullet, S. Massart, S. Collini, G. Pieraccini, and P. Lionetti. "Impact of Diet in Shaping Gut Microbiota Revealed by a Comparative Study in Children from Europe and Rural Africa." Proceedings of the National Academy of Sciences 107, no. 33 (August 02, 2010): 14691-4696. http://www.ncbi.nlm.nih.gov/pmc/articles/ PMC2930426/.

50. O'Keefe, Stephen J. D., Jia V. Li, Leo Lahti, Junhai Ou, Franck Carbonero, Khaled Mohammed, Joram M. Posma, James Kinross, Elaine Wahl, Elizabeth Ruder, Kishore Vipperla, Vasudevan Naidoo, Lungile Mtshali, Sebastian Tims, Philippe G. B. Puylaert, James Delany, Alyssa Krasinskas, Ann C. Benefiel, Hatem O. Kaseb, Keith Newton, Jeremy K. Nicholson, Willem M. De Vos, H. Rex Gaskins, and Erwin G. Zoetendal. "Fat, Fibre and Cancer Risk in African Americans and Rural Africans." Nature Communications Nat Comms 6 (April 28, 2015): 6342. http://www.ncbi.nlm.nih.gov/ pmc/articles/PMC4415091/.

51. Fung, Teresa T. "Low-Carbohydrate Diets and All-Cause and Cause-Specific Mortality." Annals of Internal Medicine Ann Intern Med 153, no. 5 (September 07, 2010): 289. http://www.ncbi.nlm.nih.gov/ pubmed/20820038.

52. Galeone, C., C. Pelucchi, F. Levi, E. Negri, S. Franceschi, R. Talamini, A. Giacosa, and C. La Vecchia. "Result Filters." National Center for Biotechnology Information. November 2006. http://www. ncbi.nlm.nih.gov/pubmed/17093154.

53. Chang, Hye-Sook, Osamu Yamato, Masahiro Yamasaki, Miyan Ko, and Yoshimitsu Maede. "Growth Inhibitory Effect of Alk(en)yl Thiosulfates Derived from Onion and Garlic in Human Immortalized and Tumor Cell Lines." Cancer Letters 223, no. 1 (June 1, 2005): 47-55. http://www.ncbi.nlm.nih.gov/pubmed/15890236.

54. Block, Eric. "Organoselenium and Organosulfur Phytochemicals

from Genus Allium Plants (Onion, Garlic): Relevance for Cancer Protection." Food Factors for Cancer Prevention, 1997, 215-21. http://link.springer.com/chapter/10.1007/978-4-431-67017-9_43.

55. Seki, Taiichiro, Kentaro Tsuji, Yumi Hayato, Tadaaki Moritomo, and Toyohiko Ariga. "Garlic and Onion Oils Inhibit Proliferation and Induce Differentiation of HL-60 Cells." Cancer Letters 160, no. 1 (November 10, 2000): 29-35. http://www.ncbi.nlm.nih.gov/pubmed/11098081.

56. Ariga, Toyohiko, and Taiichiro Seki. "Antithrombotic and Anticancer Effects of Garlic-derived Sulfur Compounds: A Review." BioFactors 26, no. 2 (2006): 93-103. http://www.ncbi.nlm.nih.gov/pubmed/16823096.

57. Nicastro, H. L., S. A. Ross, and J. A. Milner. "Garlic and Onions: Their Cancer Prevention Properties." Cancer Prevention Research 8, no. 3 (January 13, 2015): 181-89. http://www.ncbi.nlm.nih.gov/pubmed/25586902.

58. Tsubura, Airo, Yen-Chang Lai, Maki Kuwata, Norihisa Uehara, and Katsuhiko Yoshizawa. "Anticancer Effects of Garlic and Garlic-derived Compounds for Breast Cancer Control." Anti-Cancer Agents in Medicinal Chemistry ACAMC 11, no. 3 (March 2011): 249-53. http://www.ncbi.nlm.nih.gov/pubmed/21269259.

59. Zhou, Yong, Wen Zhuang, Wen Hu, Guan–Jian Liu, Tai–Xiang Wu, and Xiao–Ting Wu. "Consumption of Large Amounts of Allium Vegetables Reduces Risk for Gastric Cancer in a Meta-analysis." Gastroenterology 141, no. 1 (April 5, 2011): 80-89. http://www.ncbi.nlm.nih.gov/pubmed/21473867.

60. Mahabir, S. "Dietary Fiber Intake and Risk of Breast Cancer: A Meta-analysis of Prospective Cohort Studies." Breast Diseases: A Year Book Quarterly 23, no. 1 (September 2011): 29-30. http://www.ncbi.nlm.nih.gov/pubmed/21775566.

61. Pierini, Roberto, Jennifer M. Gee, Nigel J. Belshaw, and Ian T. Johnson. "Flavonoids and Intestinal Cancers." BJN British Journal of Nutrition 99, no. E-S1 (May 2008). http://www.ncbi.nlm.nih.gov/pubmed/18503735.

62. Li, Jiaoyuan, Li Zou, Wei Chen, Beibei Zhu, Na Shen, Juntao Ke,

Jiao Lou, Ranran Song, Rong Zhong, and Xiaoping Miao. "Dietary Mushroom Intake May Reduce the Risk of Breast Cancer: Evidence from a Meta-Analysis of Observational Studies." PLoS ONE 9, no. 4 (April 01, 2014). http://journals.plos.org/plosone/article?id=10.1371/journal.pone.0093437.

63. Martin, K. R., and S. K. Brophy. "Commonly Consumed and Specialty Dietary Mushrooms Reduce Cellular Proliferation in MCF-7 Human Breast Cancer Cells." Experimental Biology and Medicine 235, no. 11 (November 2010): 1306-314. http://www.ncbi.nlm.nih.gov/pubmed/20921274.

64. Fang, Nianbai, Qinglin Li, Shanggong Yu, Jianxiang Zhang, Ling He, Martin J.j. Ronis, and Thomas M. Badger. "Inhibition of Growth and Induction of Apoptosis in Human Cancer Cell Lines by an Ethyl Acetate Fraction from Shiitake Mushrooms." The Journal of Alternative and Complementary Medicine 12, no. 2 (March 2006): 125-32. http://www.ncbi.nlm.nih.gov/pubmed/16566671.

65. Shin, Aesun, Jeongseon Kim, Sun-Young Lim, Gaeul Kim, Mi-Kyung Sung, Eun-Sook Lee, and Jungsil Ro. "Dietary Mushroom Intake and the Risk of Breast Cancer Based on Hormone Receptor Status." Nutrition and Cancer 62, no. 4 (2010): 476-83. http://www.ncbi.nlm.nih.gov/pubmed/20432168.

66. Stoner, G. D., L.-S. Wang, and B. C. Casto. "Laboratory and Clinical Studies of Cancer Chemoprevention by Antioxidants in Berries." Carcinogenesis 29, no. 9 (June 09, 2008): 1665-674. http://www.ncbi.nlm.nih.gov/pubmed/18544560.

67. Jaganathan, Saravana Kumar. "Chemopreventive Effect of Apple and Berry Fruits against Colon Cancer." World Journal of Gastroenterology WJG 20, no. 45 (December 7, 2014): 17029. http://www.ncbi.nlm.nih.gov/pmc/articles/PMC4258571/.

68. Hannum, Sandra M. "Potential Impact of Strawberries on Human Health: A Review of the Science." Critical Reviews in Food Science and Nutrition 44, no. 1 (2004): 1-17. http://www.ncbi.nlm.nih.gov/pubmed/15077879.

69. Wang, Shiow Y. "Correlation of Antioxidants and Antioxidant Enzymes to Oxygen Radical Scavenging Activities in Berries." Berries and Cancer Prevention, November 12, 2010, 79-97. http://link.

springer.com/chapter/10.1007/978-1-4419-7554-6_4.

70. Yang, Allison, Haonan Li, Wanying Zhang, Yeon Tae Chung, Jie Liao, and Guang-Yu Yang. "Chemoprevention of Chronic Inflammatory Bowel Disease-Induced Carcinogenesis in Rodent Models by Berries." Berries and Cancer Prevention, November 12, 2010, 227-43. http://link.springer.com/chapter/10.1007/978-1-4419-7554-6_12.

71. Afaq, Farrukh. "Botanical Antioxidants for Chemoprevention of Photocarcinogenesis." Frontiers in Bioscience Front Biosci 7, no. 1-3 (April 2002): D784. http://www.ncbi.nlm.nih.gov/pubmed/11897547.

72. Afaq, Farrukh, and Hasan Mukhtar. "Botanical Antioxidants in the Prevention of Photocarcinogenesis and Photoaging." Experimental Dermatology Exp Dermatol 15, no. 9 (September 2006): 678-84. http://www.ncbi.nlm.nih.gov/pubmed/16881964.

73. Roy, Sashwati, Savita Khanna, Helaine M. Alessio, Jelena Vider, Debasis Bagchi, Manashi Bagchi, and Chandan K. Sen. "Anti-angiogenic Property of Edible Berries." Free Radical Research 36, no. 9 (September 2002): 1023-032. http://www.ncbi.nlm.nih.gov/pubmed/12448828.

74. Khan, N., F. Afaq, M.-H. Kweon, K. Kim, and H. Mukhtar. "Oral Consumption of Pomegranate Fruit Extract Inhibits Growth and Progression of Primary Lung Tumors in Mice." Cancer Research 67, no. 7 (April 01, 2007): 3475-482. http://www.ncbi.nlm.nih.gov/pubmed/17389758.

75. Sartippour, Maryam, Navindra Seeram, Jian Rao, Aune Moro, Diane Harris, Susanne Henning, Amita Firouzi, Matthew Rettig, William Aronson, Allan Pantuck, and David Heber. "Ellagitannin-rich Pomegranate Extract Inhibits Angiogenesis in Prostate Cancer in Vitro and in Vivo." Int J Oncol International Journal of Oncology, February 2008. http://www.ncbi.nlm.nih.gov/pubmed/18202771.

76. Thompson, L. U. "Dietary Flaxseed Alters Tumor Biological Markers in Postmenopausal Breast Cancer." Clinical Cancer Research 11, no. 10 (May 15, 2005): 3828-835. http://www.ncbi.nlm.nih.gov/pubmed/15897583.

77. Meadows, Gary G. "Diet, Nutrients, Phytochemicals, and Cancer

Metastasis Suppressor Genes." Cancer Metastasis Rev Cancer and Metastasis Reviews 31, no. 3-4 (December 2012): 441-54. http://www.ncbi.nlm.nih.gov/pubmed/22692480.

78. Singh, B. N., Harikesh Bahadur Singh, A. Singh, Alim H. Naqvi, and Braj Raj Singh. "Dietary Phytochemicals Alter Epigenetic Events and Signaling Pathways for Inhibition of Metastasis Cascade." Cancer Metastasis Rev Cancer and Metastasis Reviews 33, no. 1 (March 2014): 41-85. http://www.ncbi.nlm.nih.gov/pubmed/24390421.

79. Lee, Jong Hun, Tin Oo Khor, Limin Shu, Zheng-Yuan Su, Francisco Fuentes, and Ah-Ng Tony Kong. "Dietary Phytochemicals and Cancer Prevention: Nrf2 Signaling, Epigenetics, and Cell Death Mechanisms in Blocking Cancer Initiation and Progression." Pharmacology & Therapeutics 137, no. 2 (February 2013): 153-71. http://www.ncbi.nlm.nih.gov/pubmed/23041058.

80. Gopalakrishnan, Avanthika, and Ah-Ng Tony Kong. "Anticarcinogenesis by Dietary Phytochemicals: Cytoprotection by Nrf2 in Normal Cells and Cytotoxicity by Modulation of Transcription Factors NF-κB and AP-1 in Abnormal Cancer Cells." Food and Chemical Toxicology 46, no. 4 (September 15, 2007): 1257-270. http://www.ncbi.nlm.nih.gov/pubmed/17950513.

81. Lam, T. K., L. Gallicchio, K. Lindsley, M. Shiels, E. Hammond, X. Tao, L. Chen, K. A. Robinson, L. E. Caulfield, J. G. Herman, E. Guallar, and A. J. Alberg. "Cruciferous Vegetable Consumption and Lung Cancer Risk: A Systematic Review." Cancer Epidemiology Biomarkers & Prevention 18, no. 1 (January 2009): 184-95. http://www.ncbi.nlm.nih.gov/pubmed/19124497.

82. Wu, Xiang, Qing-Hua Zhou, and Ke Xu. "Are Isothiocyanates Potential Anti-cancer Drugs?" Acta Pharmacologica Sinica Acta Pharmacol Sin 30, no. 5 (2009): 501-12. http://www.nature.com/aps/journal/v30/n5/full/aps200950a.html.

83. Wu, Qi-Jun, Yang Yang, Jing Wang, Li-Hua Han, and Yong-Bing Xiang. "Cruciferous Vegetable Consumption and Gastric Cancer Risk: A Meta-analysis of Epidemiological Studies." Cancer Science Cancer Sci 104, no. 8 (August 2013): 1067-073. http://www.ncbi.nlm.nih.gov/pubmed/23679348.

84. Tse, Genevieve, and Guy D. Eslick. "Cruciferous Vegetables and Risk

of Colorectal Neoplasms: A Systematic Review and Meta-Analysis." Nutrition and Cancer 66, no. 1 (December 16, 2013): 128-39. http://www.ncbi.nlm.nih.gov/pubmed/24341734.

85. Tang, Li, Gary R. Zirpoli, Vijayvel Jayaprakash, Mary E. Reid, Susan E. Mccann, Chukwumere E. Nwogu, Yuesheng Zhang, Christine B. Ambrosone, and Kirsten B. Moysich. "Cruciferous Vegetable Intake Is Inversely Associated with Lung Cancer Risk among Smokers: A Case-control Study." BMC Cancer 10, no. 1 (April 27, 2010): 162. http://www.ncbi.nlm.nih.gov/pubmed/20423504.

86. Li, Li-Yi, Yue Luo, Ming-Dong Lu, Xiao-Wu Xu, Hai-Duo Lin, and Zhi-Qiang Zheng. "Cruciferous Vegetable Consumption and the Risk of Pancreatic Cancer: A Meta-analysis." World J Surg Onc World Journal of Surgical Oncology 13, no. 1 (February 12, 2015): 44. http://www.ncbi.nlm.nih.gov/pmc/articles/PMC4336706/.

87. Scarpa, Emanuele-Salvatore, and Paolino Ninfali. "Phytochemicals as Innovative Therapeutic Tools against Cancer Stem Cells." IJMS International Journal of Molecular Sciences 16, no. 7 (July 10, 2015): 15727-5742. http://www.mdpi.com/1422-0067/16/7/15727/htm.

88. Phillips, J., T. Moore-Medlin, K. Sonavane, O. Ekshyyan, J. Mclarty, and C.-A. O. Nathan. "Curcumin Inhibits UV Radiation-Induced Skin Cancer in SKH-1 Mice." Otolaryngology -- Head and Neck Surgery 148, no. 5 (May 2013): 797-803. http://www.ncbi.nlm.nih. gov/pubmed/23386626.

89. Osterman, Carlos J. Diaz, James C. Lynch, Patrick Leaf, Amber Gonda, Heather R. Ferguson Bennit, Duncan Griffiths, and Nathan R. Wall. "Curcumin Modulates Pancreatic Adenocarcinoma Cell-Derived Exosomal Function." PLOS ONE PLoS ONE 10, no. 7 (July 15, 2015). http://www.ncbi.nlm.nih.gov/pubmed/26177391.

90. Taverna, Simona, Marco Giallombardo, Marzia Pucci, Anna Flugy, Mauro Manno, Samuele Raccosta, Christian Rolfo, Giacomo De Leo, and Riccardo Alessandro. "Curcumin Inhibits in Vitro and in Vivo Chronic Myelogenous Leukemia Cells Growth: A Possible Role for Exosomal Disposal of MiR-21." Oncotarget 6, no. 26 (September 8, 2015): 21918-1933. http://www.ncbi.nlm.nih.gov/ pubmed/26116834.

91. Zhang, Huang-Ge, Helen Kim, Cunren Liu, Shaohua Yu, Jianhua

Wang, William E. Grizzle, Robert P. Kimberly, and Stephen Barnes. "Curcumin Reverses Breast Tumor Exosomes Mediated Immune Suppression of NK Cell Tumor Cytotoxicity." Biochimica Et Biophysica Acta (BBA) - Molecular Cell Research 1773, no. 7 (May 1, 2007): 1116-123. http://www.ncbi.nlm.nih.gov/pubmed/17555831.

92. Zhao, Zhiming, Chenggang Li, Hao Xi, Yuanxing Gao, and Dabin Xu. "Curcumin Induces Apoptosis in Pancreatic Cancerï¿½cells through the Induction of Forkhead Box O1 and Inhibition of the PI3K/Akt Pathway." Molecular Medicine Reports Mol Med Report, July 08, 2015. http://www.ncbi.nlm.nih.gov/pubmed/26166196.

93. Li, Zhen-Cai, Li-Ming Zhang, Hai-Bin Wang, Jun-Xun Ma, and Jun-Zhong Sun. "Curcumin Inhibits Lung Cancer Progression and Metastasis through Induction of FOXO1." Tumor Biol. Tumor Biology 35, no. 1 (July 26, 2013): 111-16. http://www.ncbi.nlm.nih.gov/pubmed/23888319.

94. Kunnumakkara, Ajaikumar B., Preetha Anand, and Bharat B. Aggarwal. "Curcumin Inhibits Proliferation, Invasion, Angiogenesis and Metastasis of Different Cancers through Interaction with Multiple Cell Signaling Proteins." Cancer Letters 269, no. 2 (May 13, 2008): 199-225. http://www.ncbi.nlm.nih.gov/pubmed/18479807.

95. Dhandapani, Krishnan M., Virendra B. Mahesh, and Darrell W. Brann. "Curcumin Suppresses Growth and Chemoresistance of Human Glioblastoma Cells via AP-1 and NFκB Transcription Factors." Journal of Neurochemistry 102, no. 2 (July 2007): 522-38. http://www.ncbi.nlm.nih.gov/pubmed/17596214.

96. Bush, Jason A., K-John J. Cheung, and Gang Li. "Curcumin Induces Apoptosis in Human Melanoma Cells through a Fas Receptor/Caspase-8 Pathway Independent of P53." Experimental Cell Research 271, no. 2 (December 10, 2001): 305-14. http://www.ncbi.nlm.nih.gov/pubmed/11716543.

97. Jiang, Ai-Jun, Guan Jiang, Lian-Tao Li, and Jun-Nian Zheng. "Curcumin Induces Apoptosis through Mitochondrial Pathway and Caspases Activation in Human Melanoma Cells." Molecular Biology Reports Mol Biol Rep 42, no. 1 (September 28, 2014): 267-75. Curcumin induces apoptosis through mitochondrial pathway and

caspases activation in human melanoma cells.

98. Schäfer, Georgia, and Catherine Kaschula. "The Immunomodulation and Anti-Inflammatory Effects of Garlic Organosulfur Compounds in Cancer Chemoprevention." Anti-Cancer Agents in Medicinal Chemistry ACAMC 14, no. 2 (February 2014): 233-40. http://www.ncbi.nlm.nih.gov/pubmed/24237225.

99. Nagini, Siddavaram. "Cancer Chemoprevention by Garlic and Its Organosulfur Compounds-Panacea or Promise?" Anti-Cancer Agents in Medicinal Chemistry ACAMC 8, no. 3 (April 2008): 313-21. http://www.ncbi.nlm.nih.gov/pubmed/18393790.

100. Cerella, Claudia, Mario Dicato, Claus Jacob, and Marc Diederich. "Chemical Properties and Mechanisms Determining the Anti-Cancer Action of Garlic-Derived Organic Sulfur Compounds." Anti-Cancer Agents in Medicinal Chemistry ACAMC 11, no. 3 (March 2011): 267-71. http://www.ncbi.nlm.nih.gov/pubmed/21269260.

101. Jin, Z.-Y., M. Wu, R.-Q. Han, X.-F. Zhang, X.-S. Wang, A.-M. Liu, J.-Y. Zhou, Q.-Y. Lu, Z.-F. Zhang, and J.-K. Zhao. "Raw Garlic Consumption as a Protective Factor for Lung Cancer, a Population-Based Case-Control Study in a Chinese Population." Cancer Prevention Research 6, no. 7 (May 08, 2013): 711-18. CLPTM1L polymorphism as a protective factor for lung cancer: a case–control study in southern Chinese population.

102. Gao, Chang-Ming, Kazuo Tajima, Tetsuo Kuroishi, Kaoru Hirose, and Manami Inoue. "Protective Effects of Raw Vegetables and Fruit against Lung Cancer among Smokers and Ex-smokers: A Case-Control Study in the Tokai Area of Japan." Japanese Journal of Cancer Research 84, no. 6 (June 1993): 594-600. http://www.ncbi.nlm.nih.gov/pubmed/8340248.

103. Al-Menhali, Afnan, Aisha Al-Rumaihi, Hana Al-Mohammed, Hana Al-Mazrooey, Maryam Al-Shamlan, Meaad Aljassim, Noof Al-Korbi, and Ali Hussein Eid. "Thymus Vulgaris (Thyme) Inhibits Proliferation, Adhesion, Migration, and Invasion of Human Colorectal Cancer Cells." Journal of Medicinal Food 18, no. 1 (January 2015): 54-59. http://www.ncbi.nlm.nih.gov/pubmed/25379783.

104. Galasso, Silvia, Severina Pacifico, Nadine Kretschmer, San-Po Pan,

Sabina Marciano, Simona Piccolella, Pietro Monaco, and Rudolf Bauer. "Influence of Seasonal Variation on Thymus Longicaulis C. Presl Chemical Composition and Its Antioxidant and Anti-inflammatory Properties." Phytochemistry 107 (September 16, 2014): 80-90. http://www.ncbi.nlm.nih.gov/pubmed/25239551.

105. Qi, Lian-Wen, Zhiyu Zhang, Chun-Feng Zhang, Samantha Anderson, Qun Liu, Chun-Su Yuan, and Chong-Zhi Wang. "Anti-Colon Cancer Effects of 6-Shogaol Through G2/M Cell Cycle Arrest by P53/p21-cdc2/cdc25A Crosstalk." The American Journal of Chinese Medicine Am. J. Chin. Med. 43, no. 04 (June 28, 2015): 743-56. http://www.ncbi.nlm.nih.gov/pubmed/26119958.

106. Akimoto, Miho, Mari Iizuka, Rie Kanematsu, Masato Yoshida, and Keizo Takenaga. "Anticancer Effect of Ginger Extract against Pancreatic Cancer Cells Mainly through Reactive Oxygen Species-Mediated Autotic Cell Death." PLOS ONE PLoS ONE 10, no. 5 (May 11, 2015). http://www.ncbi.nlm.nih.gov/pubmed/25961833.

107. Han, Min Ae, Seon Min Woo, Kyoung-Jin Min, Shin Kim, Jong-Wook Park, Dong Eun Kim, Sang Hyun Kim, Yung Hyun Choi, and Taeg Kyu Kwon. "6-Shogaol Enhances Renal Carcinoma Caki Cells to TRAIL-induced Apoptosis through Reactive Oxygen Species-mediated Cytochrome C Release and Down-regulation of C-FLIP(L) Expression." Chemico-Biological Interactions 228 (February 25, 2015): 69-78. http://www.ncbi.nlm.nih.gov/pubmed/25619640.

108. Poltronieri, Juliana, Amanda Becceneri, Angelina Fuzer, Julio Filho, Ana Martin, Paulo Vieira, Normand Pouliot, and Márcia Cominetti. "[6]-gingerol as a Cancer Chemopreventive Agent: A Review of Its Activity on Different Steps of the Metastatic Process." MRMC Mini-Reviews in Medicinal Chemistry 14, no. 4 (April 2014): 313-21. http://www.ncbi.nlm.nih.gov/pubmed/24552266.

109. Radhakrishnan, Ek, Smitha V. Bava, Sai Shyam Narayanan, Lekshmi R. Nath, Arun Kumar T. Thulasidasan, Eppurathu Vasudevan Soniya, and Ruby JohnAnto. "[6]-Gingerol Induces Caspase-Dependent Apoptosis and Prevents PMA-Induced Proliferation in Colon Cancer Cells by Inhibiting MAPK/AP-1 Signaling." PLoS ONE 9, no. 8 (August 26, 2014). http://www.ncbi.nlm.nih.gov/pubmed/25157570.

110. Ryu, Min Ju, and Ha Sook Chung. "[10]-Gingerol Induces

Mitochondrial Apoptosis through Activation of MAPK Pathway in HCT116 Human Colon Cancer Cells." In Vitro Cellular & Developmental Biology - Animal In Vitro Cell.Dev.Biol.-Animal 51, no. 1 (August 23, 2014): 92-101. http://www.ncbi.nlm.nih.gov/pubmed/25148824.

111. Yuan, Chun-Su. "Genistein Induces G2/M Cell Cycle Arrest and Apoptosis via ATM/p53-dependent Pathway in Human Colon Cancer Cells." Int J Oncol International Journal of Oncology, May 17, 2013. http://www.ncbi.nlm.nih.gov/pubmed/23686257.

112. Varinska, Lenka, Peter Gal, Gabriela Mojzisova, Ladislav Mirossay, and Jan Mojzis. "Soy and Breast Cancer: Focus on Angiogenesis." IJMS International Journal of Molecular Sciences 16, no. 5 (May 22, 2015): 11728-1749. http://www.ncbi.nlm.nih.gov/pubmed/26006245.

113. Mahmoud, Abeer M., Wancai Yang, and Maarten C. Bosland. "Soy Isoflavones and Prostate Cancer: A Review of Molecular Mechanisms." The Journal of Steroid Biochemistry and Molecular Biology 140 (March 2014): 116-32. http://www.ncbi.nlm.nih.gov/pubmed/24373791.

114. Hsu, A., T. M. Bray, W. G. Helferich, D. R. Doerge, and E. Ho. "Differential Effects of Whole Soy Extract and Soy Isoflavones on Apoptosis in Prostate Cancer Cells." Experimental Biology and Medicine 235, no. 1 (January 2010): 90-97. http://www.ncbi.nlm.nih.gov/pubmed/20404023.

115. Adjakly, Mawussi, Marejolaine Ngollo, Jean-Paul Boiteux, Yves-Jean Bignon, Laurent Guy, and Dominique Bernard-Gallon. "Genistein and Daidzein: Different Molecular Effects on Prostate Cancer." Genistein and Daidzein: Different Molecular Effects on Prostate Cancer. January 2013. http://ar.iiarjournals.org/content/33/1/39.long.

116. Sarkar, Fazlul H., and Yiwei Li. "Soy Isoflavones and Cancer Prevention." Cancer Investigation 21, no. 5 (2003): 744-57. http://www.ncbi.nlm.nih.gov/pubmed/14628433.

117. Ouyang, Gaoliang, Luming Yao, Kai Ruan, Gang Song, Yubin Mao, and Shideng Bao. "Genistein Induces G2/M Cell Cycle Arrest and Apoptosis of Human Ovarian Cancer Cells via Activation of DNA

Damage Checkpoint Pathways." Cell Biology International 33, no. 12 (September 2, 2009): 1237-244. http://www.ncbi.nlm.nih.gov/pubmed/19732843.

118. Ismail, Ismail Ahmed, Ku-Seong Kang, Hae Ahm Lee, Jung-Wan Kim, and Yoon-Kyung Sohn. "Genistein-induced Neuronal Apoptosis and G2/M Cell Cycle Arrest Is Associated with MDC1 Up-regulation and PLK1 Down-regulation." European Journal of Pharmacology 575, no. 1-3 (July 28, 2007): 12-20. http://www.ncbi.nlm.nih.gov/pubmed/17706963.

119. Die, M. Diana Van, Kerry M. Bone, Scott G. Williams, and Marie V. Pirotta. "Soy and Soy Isoflavones in Prostate Cancer: A Systematic Review and Meta-analysis of Randomized Controlled Trials." BJU International BJU Int 113, no. 5b (May 2014). http://www.ncbi.nlm.nih.gov/pubmed/24053483.

120. Dong, Xin, Wenqing Xu, Robert A. Sikes, and Changqing Wu. "Combination of Low Dose of Genistein and Daidzein Has Synergistic Preventive Effects on Isogenic Human Prostate Cancer Cells When Compared with Individual Soy Isoflavone." Food Chemistry 141, no. 3 (May 9, 2013): 1923-933. http://www.ncbi.nlm.nih.gov/pubmed/23870911.

121. Dong, Xin, Wenqing Xu, Robert A. Sikes, and Changqing Wu. "Apoptotic Effects of Cooked and in Vitro Digested Soy on Human Prostate Cancer Cells." Food Chemistry 135, no. 3 (January 26, 2012): 1643-652. http://www.ncbi.nlm.nih.gov/pubmed/22953905.

122. Pudenz, Maria, Kevin Roth, and Clarissa Gerhauser. "Impact of Soy Isoflavones on the Epigenome in Cancer Prevention." Nutrients 6, no. 10 (October 15, 2014): 4218-272. http://www.ncbi.nlm.nih.gov/pubmed/25322458.

123. Karsli-Ceppioglu, Seher, Marjolaine Ngollo, Mawussi Adjakly, Aslihan Dagdemir, Gaëlle Judes, André Lebert, Jean-Paul Boiteux, Frédérique Penault-Llorca, Yves-Jean Bignon, Laurent Guy, and Dominique Bernard-Gallon. "Genome-Wide DNA Methylation Modified by Soy Phytoestrogens: Role for Epigenetic Therapeutics in Prostate Cancer?" OMICS: A Journal of Integrative Biology 19, no. 4 (April 2015): 209-19. http://www.ncbi.nlm.nih.gov/pubmed/25831061.

REFERENCES

124. Adjakly, Mawussi, Marjolaine Ngollo, Aslihan Dagdemir, Gaëlle Judes, Amaury Pajon, Seher Karsli-Ceppioglu, Frédérique Penault-Llorca, Jean-Paul Boiteux, Yves-Jean Bignon, Laurent Guy, and Dominique Bernard-Gallon. "Prostate Cancer: The Main Risk and Protective Factors – Epigenetic Modifications." Annales D'Endocrinologie 76, no. 1 (January 13, 2015): 25-41. http://www.ncbi.nlm.nih.gov/pubmed/25592466.

125. Vardi, A., R. Bosviel, N. Rabiau, M. Adjakly, S. Satih, P. Dechelotte, J. P. Boiteux, L. Fontana, Y. J. Bignon, L. Guy, and D. J. Bernard-Gallon. "Soy Phytoestrogens Modify DNA Methylation of GSTP1, RASSF1A, EPH2 and BRCA1 Promoter in Prostate Cancer Cells." National Center for Biotechnology Information. July/August 2010. http://www.ncbi.nlm.nih.gov/pubmed/20668305.

126. Bosviel, Rémy, Elise Dumollard, Pierre Déchelotte, Yves-Jean Bignon, and Dominique Bernard-Gallon. "Can Soy Phytoestrogens Decrease DNA Methylation in BRCA1 and BRCA2 Oncosuppressor Genes in Breast Cancer?" OMICS: A Journal of Integrative Biology 16, no. 5 (February 17, 2012): 235-44. http://www.ncbi.nlm.nih.gov/pubmed/22339411.

127. Bernard-Gallon, D. J., S. Satih, N. Chalabi, N. Rabiau, R. Bosviel, L. Fontana, and Y. J. Bignon. "Phytoestrogens Regulate the Expression of Genes Involved in Different Biological Processes in BRCA2 Knocked down MCF-7, MDA-MB-231 and MCF-10a Cell Lines." Oncology Reports Oncol Rep 23, no. 3 (March 2010). http://www.ncbi.nlm.nih.gov/pubmed/20127002.

128. Suboj, Priya, Suboj Babykutty, Priya Srinivas, and Srinivas Gopala. "Aloe Emodin Induces G2/M Cell Cycle Arrest and Apoptosis via Activation of Caspase-6 in Human Colon Cancer Cells." Pharmacology 89, no. 1-2 (February 14, 2012): 91-98. http://www.ncbi.nlm.nih.gov/pubmed/22343391.

129. Lin, Meng-Liang, Yao-Cheng Lu, Jing-Gung Chung, Yi-Chen Li, Shyang-Guang Wang, Sue-Hwee Ng, Chia-Yin Wu, Hong-Lin Su, and Shih-Shun Chen. "Aloe-emodin Induces Apoptosis of Human Nasopharyngeal Carcinoma Cells via Caspase-8-mediated Activation of the Mitochondrial Death Pathway." Cancer Letters 291, no. 1 (May 1, 2010): 46-58. http://www.ncbi.nlm.nih.gov/

pubmed/19942342.

130. Chen, Ruie, Jinming Zhang, Yangyang Hu, Shengpeng Wang, Meiwan Chen, and Yitao Wang. "Potential Antineoplastic Effects of Aloe-emodin: A Comprehensive Review." The American Journal of Chinese Medicine Am. J. Chin. Med. 42, no. 02 (2014): 275-88. http://www.ncbi.nlm.nih.gov/pubmed/24707862.

131. Jeon, Won, Young Keul Jeon, and Myeong Jin Nam. "Apoptosis by Aloe-emodin Is Mediated through Down-regulation of Calpain-2 and Ubiquitin-protein Ligase E3A in Human Hepatoma Huh-7 Cells." Cell. Biol. Int. Cell Biology International 36, no. 2 (February 2012): 163-67. http://www.ncbi.nlm.nih.gov/pubmed/21861846.

132. El-Shemy, H., M. Aboul-Soud, A. Nassr-Allah, K. Aboul-Enein, A. Kabash, and A. Yagi. "Antitumor Properties and Modulation of Antioxidant Enzymes Activity by Aloe Vera Leaf Active Principles Isolated via Supercritical Carbon Dioxide Extraction." CMC Current Medicinal Chemistry 17, no. 2 (2010): 129-38. http://www.ncbi.nlm.nih.gov/pubmed/19941474.

133. Lee, Keyong Ho, Jeong Hwan Kim, Dae Seog Lim, and Chang Han Kim. "Anti-leukaemic and Anti-mutagenic Effects of Di(2-ethylhexyl) phthalate Isolated FromAloe VeraLinne." Journal of Pharmacy and Pharmacology 52, no. 5 (May 2000): 593-98. http://www.ncbi.nlm.nih.gov/pubmed/10864149.

134. Tyagi, Alpna, Komal Raina, Subhash Gangar, Manjinder Kaur, Rajesh Agarwal, and Chapla Agarwal. "Differential Effect of Grape Seed Extract against Human Non-small-Cell Lung Cancer Cells: The Role of Reactive Oxygen Species and Apoptosis Induction." Nutrition and Cancer 65, no. Sup1 (2013): 44-53. http://www.ncbi.nlm.nih.gov/pubmed/23682782.

135. Shrotriya, Sangeeta, Gagan Deep, Mallikarjuna Gu, Manjinder Kaur, Anil K. Jain, Swetha Inturi, Rajesh Agarwal, and Chapla Agarwal. "Abstract 1598: Grape Seed Extract Induces Irreparable DNA Damage Causing G2/M Arrest and Apoptosis Selectively in Head and Neck Squamous Cell Carcinoma Cells: Potential Involvement of Reactive Oxygen Species." Cancer Research Cancer Res 72, no. 8 Supplement (2012): 1598. http://cancerres.aacrjournals.org/content/72/8_Supplement/1598.short.

136. Dinicola, Simona, Maria Addolorata Mariggiò, Caterina Morabito, Simone |Guarnieri, Alessandra Cucina, Alessia Pasqualato, Fabrizio D'anselmi, Sara Proietti, Pierpaolo Coluccia, and Mariano Bizzarri. "Grape Seed Extract Triggers Apoptosis in Caco-2 Human Colon Cancer Cells through Reactive Oxygen Species and Calcium Increase: Extracellular Signal-regulated Kinase Involvement." British Journal of Nutrition Br J Nutr 110, no. 05 (February 25, 2013): 797-809. http://www.ncbi.nlm.nih.gov/pubmed/23433299.

137. Derry, M. M., K. Raina, V. Balaiya, A. K. Jain, S. Shrotriya, K. M. Huber, N. J. Serkova, R. Agarwal, and C. Agarwal. "Grape Seed Extract Efficacy against Azoxymethane-Induced Colon Tumorigenesis in A/J Mice: Interlinking MiRNA with Cytokine Signaling and Inflammation." Cancer Prevention Research 6, no. 7 (May 02, 2013): 625-33. http://www.ncbi.nlm.nih.gov/pubmed/23639480.

138. Derry, Molly M., Komal Raina, Rajesh Agarwal, and Chapla Agarwal. "Characterization of Azoxymethane-induced Colon Tumor Metastasis to Lung in a Mouse Model Relevant to Human Sporadic Colorectal Cancer and Evaluation of Grape Seed Extract Efficacy." Experimental and Toxicologic Pathology 66, no. 5-6 (March 23, 2014): 235-42. http://www.ncbi.nlm.nih.gov/pubmed/24670932.

139. Raina, Komal, Alpna Tyagi, Dileep Kumar, Rajesh Agarwal, and Chapla Agarwal. "Role of Oxidative Stress in Cytotoxicity of Grape Seed Extract in Human Bladder Cancer Cells." Food and Chemical Toxicology 61 (July 3, 2013): 187-95. http://www.ncbi.nlm.nih.gov/pubmed/23831192.

140. Kaur, M., C. Agarwal, and R. Agarwal. "Anticancer and Cancer Chemopreventive Potential of Grape Seed Extract and Other Grape-Based Products." Journal of Nutrition 139, no. 9 (September 2009). http://www.ncbi.nlm.nih.gov/pmc/articles/PMC2728696/.

141. Kim, Do-Hee, Ki-Woong Park, In Gyeong Chae, Juthika Kundu, Eun-Hee Kim, Joydeb Kumar Kundu, and Kyung-Soo Chun. "Carnosic Acid Inhibits STAT3 Signaling and Induces Apoptosis through Generation of ROS in Human Colon Cancer HCT116 Cells." Mol. Carcinog. Molecular Carcinogenesis, July 8, 2015. http://www.ncbi.nlm.nih.gov/pubmed/26152521.

142. Chun, Kyung-Soo. "Carnosol Induces Apoptosis through Generation

of ROS and Inactivation of STAT3 Signaling in Human Colon Cancer HCT116 Cells." Int J Oncol International Journal of Oncology, January 27, 2014. http://www.ncbi.nlm.nih.gov/pubmed/24481553.

143. Park, Ji, Byoungduck Park, In Chae, Do-Hee Kim, Juthika Kundu, Joydeb Kundu, and Kyung-Soo Chun. "Carnosic Acid Induces Apoptosis through Inactivation of Src/STAT3 Signaling Pathway in Human Renal Carcinoma Caki Cells." Oncology Reports Oncol Rep, February 29, 2016. http://www.ncbi.nlm.nih.gov/pubmed/26936454.

144. Min, Kyoung-Jin, Kyong-Jin Jung, and Taeg Kyu Kwon. "Carnosic Acid Induces Apoptosis Through Reactive Oxygen Species-mediated Endoplasmic Reticulum Stress Induction in Human Renal Carcinoma Caki Cells." Journal of Cancer Prevention 19, no. 3 (September 2014): 170-78. http://www.ncbi.nlm.nih.gov/pubmed/25337586.

145. Vanamala, Jairam, Lavanya Reddivari, Sridhar Radhakrishnan, and Chris Tarver. "Resveratrol Suppresses IGF-1 Induced Human Colon Cancer Cell Proliferation and Elevates Apoptosis via Suppression of IGF-1R/Wnt and Activation of P53 Signaling Pathways." BMC Cancer 10, no. 1 (May 26, 2010): 238. http://www.ncbi.nlm.nih.gov/pubmed/20504360.

146. Kang, Nam-Hee, Kyung-A. Hwang, Hye-Rim Lee, Dal-Woong Choi, and Kyung-Chul Choi. "Resveratrol Regulates the Cell Viability Promoted by 17β-estradiol or Bisphenol A via Down-regulation of the Cross-talk between Estrogen Receptor α and Insulin Growth Factor-1 Receptor in BG-1 Ovarian | Cancer Cells." Food and Chemical Toxicology 59 (June 27, 2013): 373-79. http://www.ncbi.nlm.nih.gov/pubmed/23810794.

147. Shan, Bao-En, Ming-Xia Wang, and Run-Qing Li. "Quercetin Inhibit Human SW480 Colon Cancer Growth in Association with Inhibition of Cyclin D 1 and Survivin Expression through Wnt/β-Catenin Signaling Pathway." Cancer Investigation 27, no. 6 (July 2009): 604-12. http://www.ncbi.nlm.nih.gov/pubmed/19440933.

148. Lee, Ra Ham, Jin Hyoung Cho, Young-Joo Jeon, Woong Bang, Jung-Jae Cho, Nag-Jin Choi, Kang Seok Seo, Jung-Hyun Shim,

and Jung-Il Chae. "Quercetin Induces Antiproliferative Activity Against Human Hepatocellular Carcinoma (HepG2) Cells by Suppressing Specificity Protein 1 (Sp1)." Drug Development Research Dru. Dev. Res., January 25, 2015. http://www.ncbi.nlm.nih.gov/pubmed/25619802.

149. Hales, Karen H., Sheree C. Speckman, Nawneet K. Kurrey, and Dale B. Hales. "Uncovering Molecular Events Associated with the Chemosuppressive Effects of Flaxseed: A Microarray Analysis of the Laying Hen Model of Ovarian Cancer." BMC Genomics 15, no. 1 (August 24, 2014): 709. http://bmcgenomics.biomedcentral.com/articles/10.1186/1471-2164-15-709(2008): 347-56. http://www.ornishspectrum.com/wp-content/uploads/A-Very-Low-Fat-Vegan-Diet-Increases.pdf.

www.ingramcontent.com/pod-product-compliance
Lightning Source LLC
Chambersburg PA
CBHW060448280326
41933CB00014B/2701